HEALING
EMOTIONS

HEALING
EMOTIONS

Conversations with the Dalai Lama on Mindfulness, Emotions, and Health

EDITED BY
DANIEL GOLEMAN, PH.D.

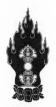

SHAMBHALA
Boston & London
1997

SHAMBHALA PUBLICATIONS, INC.
Horticultural Hall
300 Massachusetts Avenue
Boston, MA 02115
http://www.shambhala.com

9 8 7 6 5 4 3 2 1
First Edition

Printed in the United States of America

⊗ This edition is printed on acid-free paper that meets the American
National Standards Institute Z39.48 Standard.

Distributed in the United States by Random House, Inc., and in Canada by
Random House of Canada Ltd

Library of Congress Cataloging-in-Publication Data

Healing emotions: conversations with the Dalai Lama on mindfulness,
    emotions, and health/edited by Daniel Goleman.—1st ed.
      p. cm.
    Includes index.
    ISBN 1-57062-212-4 (pbk.: alk. paper)
      1. Health—Religious aspects—Buddhism.
    2. Buddhism—Psychology.   3. Buddhist ethics.
    I. Goleman, Daniel.
    BQ4570.M4H43   1997
    294.3'378321—DC21   96-47896

Contents

Acknowledgments   vii
Introduction   1

PART ONE: ETHICS
1. *Three Views of Virtue* • LEE YEARLEY   11
2. *Afflictive and Nourishing Emotions:
   Impacts on Health* • DANIEL GOLEMAN   33

PART TWO: BIOLOGICAL FOUNDATIONS
3. *The Body's Self* • FRANCISCO VARELA   49
4. *The Brain and Emotions* • CLIFF SARON
   AND RICHARD J. DAVIDSON   67
5. *Stress, Trauma, and the Body* • DANIEL
   BROWN   89

PART THREE: SKILLFUL MEANS
AND MEDICINE
6. *Mindfulness as Medicine* • SHARON
   SALZBERG AND JON KABAT-ZINN   107
7. *Behavioral Medicine* • DANIEL BROWN   145

PART FOUR: EMOTION AND CULTURE
8. *The Virtues in Christian and Buddhist
   Traditions* • LEE YEARLEY   165

9. *The Roots of Self-Esteem: Differences*
   East and West   184

PART FIVE: THE NATURE
OF AWARENESS
10. *Mind, Brain, and Body in Dialogue*   211
11. *Subtleties of Consciousness*   226

PART SIX: A UNIVERSAL ETHIC
12. *Medicine and Compassion* • THE DALAI
    LAMA   243

About the Contributors   251
Appendix   253
Index   261

ACKNOWLEDGMENTS

We are grateful for the efforts of Allan Kelley for making the first transcriptions of the Mind and Life Dialogue. Zara Houshmand did the lion's share of getting the manuscript into editable form and putting the book into its present format. Kevin and Jan Tobin offered invaluable assistance in the final stages of editing.

HEALING
EMOTIONS

INTRODUCTION

CAN THE MIND heal the body? How are the brain, immune system, and emotions interconnected? What emotions are associated with enhanced well-being? How does mindfulness function in a medical context? Is there a biological foundation for ethics? How can death help us understand the nature of the mind? In summer 1991, ten Western scholars from a broad range of diciplines gathered with the Dalai Lama in his personal meeting room in Dharamsala, India, to grapple with these questions as the focus of the third Mind and Life Conference. This book is a compendium of the presentations and dialogue that occurred at this meeting.

Experts from the fields of psychology, physiology, behavioral medicine, and philosophy presented the quintessential discoveries of their fields and discussed the connections among these findings with the Dalai Lama and with prominent practitioners of Buddhist meditation. The purpose of this cross-fertilization was to increase mutual understanding and facilitate the emergence of new insight into the relationship between health and emotional experience.

It is only in the past twenty years that Western physicians, biologists, and psychologists have begun to comprehend the interrelationship between emotional states and mental and physical well-being. Buddhist thinkers, however, have been aware of the mind's healing capacity for more than two thousand years. The presence at this conference of the foremost leader of Tibetan Buddhism provided a unique East/West synthesis. The Dalai Lama served as a touchstone for the recent scientific discoveries reported by the other participants.

THE MIND AND LIFE MEETINGS

The Dalai Lama has lived in India since he led thousands of his people to freedom from Chinese oppression in 1959. Winner of the Nobel Prize for Peace in 1989, he is universally respected as a spokesman for the compassionate and peaceful resolution of human conflict. Less well known is his intense personal interest in the sciences; he has said that if he were not a monk, he would have liked to have been an engineer. As a youth in Lhasa, it was he who was called on to fix broken machinery in the Potala Palace, be it a clock or a car.

Beginning in October 1987, the Dalai Lama has met regularly with select groups of scientists to discuss bridges and interfaces with what can broadly be called the sciences of mind and life—biology, cognitive science, neuroscience, and psychology, as well as philosophy of mind—the disciplines of most immediate relevance to the Buddhist tradition. The spirit of these meetings has been one of candor and mutual respect on both sides, as seen from the careful selection and preparation of the meetings, their private nature, the attention given to excellent translation, and the extensive time devoted to them by the Dalai Lama. The books that emerge from these dialogues—including this one, it is hoped—offer readers a sense of immediacy and spontaneity in an unprecedented exchange between a spiritual path and state-of-the-art science, between an ancient wisdom and the modern quest for answers.

BACKGROUND

This series of dialogues was initiated in 1985 jointly by Adam Engle, a U.S. attorney and businessman, and Dr. Francisco Varela, a Paris-based neurobiologist working with the National Center for Scientific Research who was aware of the importance of a serious diaolgue between science and Buddhism. The first Mind and Life Conference was held over a period of a week in Dharamsala, India, and dealt with neuroscience and cognitive science more generally. A book based on this first conference, edited by Francisco Varela and Jeremy Hayward, has been published as *Gentle Bridges: Conversations with the Dalai Lama on the Sciences of Mind* (Boston: Shambhala Publications, 1993). Since that first meeting, there have been four others, each bringing the Dalai Lama together with different groups of scientists in an atmosphere of mutual respect. Topics have included emotions and health (represented in the present volume); sleeping and dreaming, to be represented in the forthcoming book *Sleeping Dreaming and Dying* (Boston: Wisdom Publications, 1997); and the most recent conference, held in 1996, on altruism, ethics, and compassion. (For a full account of the history of the Mind and Life Conferences, see the appendix.)

Each day began with a presentation on a scientific topic, such as the neurobiology of emotions, and was followed by dialogue and debate with His Holiness, who has consistently displayed both a keen scientific mind and a breadth and depth that stretches the borders of science. For example, in this dialogue, the Dalai Lama suggests there may be subtle levels of consciousness, which Western science has yet to learn about, that do not depend on the function of the brain, unlike grosser levels that are directly related to brain activity.

An exemplar of open-minded and bold inquiry, the Dalai Lama has taken the lead in opening a dialogue between Buddhism and modern science. He sees clearly that if Tibetan Buddhism is to survive into the future, it will do so only to the degree that it is not baldly contradicted by the findings of modern scientists; he has said that if the scientific method should prove that some tenet of Buddhism is incorrect, then Buddhism would have to change accordingly.

On the other hand, the dialogues have also shown that Western science has much to gain from these insights from the East. Tibetan explorations into the psyche have yielded a sophisticated phenomenology of mind that could guide modern scientists, if scientists would listen. These dialogues are a beginning of that conversation. One fruit of these dialogues is an ongoing research project that stems directly from this third round of the Mind and Life meetings: a neurophysiological study of brain states in adept Tibetan yogis to better understand the potentials of attentional training.

Buddhism and Science, Emotions and Health: The Dialogue

Buddhism has as principal aims the goal of transforming perception and experience and synchronizing mind and body. According to Buddhist teaching, the process of harmonizing mind and body and transforming experience is a gradual one. This path is based on the practice of various forms of meditation, coupled with a moral imperative to engage in virtuous action. Such action is based on the awareness of the interdependence of all life and the universal compassion that emerges from this awareness.

Tibetan Buddhist thinkers have long been concerned with psychophysical health and have produced numerous medical treatises that date from as far back as the eleventh century. The four main Tantras (explanations) were translated from Sanskrit into Tibetan by the Lama Vairochana in the ninth century and have been handed down from teacher to student until the present day. According to this tradition, illness is the result of an imbalance in the psychophysical body which is produced by conflicting emotions such as anger or greed. Using modern experimental methods, the scientists who attended the Mind and Life Conference considered some of the same issues raised by Buddhist thinkers over the centuries.

We begin with Lee Yearley's overview of Western ethical systems and an enquiry into the possible foundations for an ethical system not based on religion. His Holiness the Dalai Lama expressed his sense of the need for such a system, which could appeal to the billions of people on the planet who hold no strong religious belief. Daniel Goleman then proposes that the workings of the body might offer such a basis, organized around which states of mind foster health and which make the body more vulnerable to disease. He reviews findings suggesting that distressing emotions can undermine health, whereas positive states may be protective.

The section on biological foundations considers some of the experimental research central to emotions and health. This section begins with a discussion on the immune system and its cognitive implications by Dr. Francisco Varela. The field of immunology is awakening to the realization that the immune system is almost a kind of "second brain," a network of specialized cells that give the body a flexible identity. Further, this somatic identity has very specific links with the neural networks underlying cognitive life, and makes up the basis of the new field of psychoneuroimmunology.

Dr. Varela's presentation, and the dialogue that accompanies it, is followed by Clifford Saron's discussion of how the brain regulates emotion. His and Richard Davidson's research elucidates how patterns of electrical activity in the brain are correlated with facial expression and other measures of mood state.

Daniel Brown's discussion of how stress affects the body details the biological foundations of the impact of emotions on health. Dr. Brown catalyzes a discussion of posttraumatic stress disorder and how it is treated; the Dalai Lama suggests that, unlike other victims of torture who then suffer from posttrauma symptoms, the experience of many Tibetans with torture by the Chinese suggests that faith and beliefs that give meaning to suffering may offer an inoculation, to some degree.

Mindfulness, a careful attention to moment-to-moment experience, is a classic Buddhist contemplative practice. Sharon Salzberg explains its basics as an introduction to the application of mindfulness in health. Cultivating beneficial emotions has a role in the treatment of disease across the medical spectrum. Jon Kabat-Zinn discusses the ways in which mindfulness meditation is being used, with good effect, to help patients develop an awareness that is less prone to being swayed by emotionality—an application of meditation practice that alleviates symptoms and facilitates healing.

Behavioral medicine uses psychological techniques to prevent or treat chronic illnesses. Daniel Brown describes how many medical symptoms are the result of physiological systems that are under stress and so out of equilibrium. State-of-the-art behavioral medicine techniques offer patients ways to regain control over the biological systems that are causing their symptoms. This new approach to healing includes modern methods such as biofeedback and ancient ones such as meditation.

In the West, psychologists readily assume pathologies of the self, especially low self-esteem, are rampant among modern humans. However, for the Dalai Lama, the very concept of low self-esteem is unknown; in Eastern cultures, where the "self" is a very different construct than in the individualistic West, there may not be such a problem. The roots of self-esteem are explored in a dialogue that suggests the self in the West may face unique problems rare in the East.

A sticking point between modern science and Buddhism is the relationship between mind and brain. Western science sees mind as an emergent property of consciousness that depends on the brain, while Tibetan Buddhist thought postulates a subtle order of consciousness not dependent on brain. Does the failure of Western science to identify mental processes that do not reduce to brain function mean there is no consciousness independent of brain? The Dalai Lama contends that extremely subtle levels of consciousness that have yet to be discovered by the West are accessible for advanced meditators, who can use them for lucid dreaming and conscious dying. If confirmed by science, such a realization would mean radically altering the paradigm of Western neuroscience.

Finally, there is a wide-ranging dialogue on the need for compassion and for an ethical system that can appeal to the billions of people who hold no particular religious faith. And so the dialogue ends with the question of whether science's new understanding of the links between mind, brain, and health might one day offer part of a basis for an ethic—guidelines for living—which upholds the values of the great world religions.

PART ONE

Ethics

WHAT THE BODY TEACHES

1

Three Views of Virtue

LEE YEARLEY

Lee Yearley introduces the conversation with a philosophical and ethical strand, one that becomes tightly woven into the deliberation as it continues. He presents an overview of three different Western philosophical traditions—individualism, perfectionism, and rationalism. Individualism asserts that what is right is what satisfies a particular individual. Rationalism proposes that for an act to be ethical, it must logically be so in all contexts. Perfectionism compares an individual's actions to a postulated ideal; the more ethical the behavior, the more it conforms to this idealized state.

Ethics in general is concerned with questions of what is right and good—that is, virtuous. But virtue depends on one's philosophical perspective. What would be considered virtuous in one system might not be in another. Dr. Yearley questions whether specific virtues such as compassion can serve as the basis for an ethical system and explains how Western philosophical thought has discarded compassion as the basis for an ethical system along with the rejection of religion. Contradictions within these Western philosophical systems are pointed out in the ensuing conversation. Dr. Yearley proposes that perfectionism, influenced by rationalism, might be the best solution for generating a universal ethical system. The Dalai Lama responds with a challenge to find a basis for moral principles that will appeal to the three or four in every five people on the planet who hold no strong religious conviction.

LEE YEARLEY: Three positions have been prevalent in the history of Western ethics.[1] Individualism bases ethics on an individual's desires. Ethics involves figuring out what you desire, then acting to get it. Perfectionism judges whether the desires an individual has are bad or good by referring to the ideal of what a perfect person is. That ideal usually rests on some notion about what human nature at its best can be. Finally, rationalism is the most distinctively modern and Western position. It claims that reason is the only proper ethical guide, defining reason to be what allows people to think about abstract universals.

A CLOSER LOOK: INDIVIDUALISM, PERFECTIONISM, RATIONALISM

Individualism never asks whether what a person wants is bad or good in some abstract sense. It only considers how best to get what a person desires. The question is not whether I should want a new Rolls Royce, but whether I can get the car, still take a vacation, and pay my therapist. Human reason has an important place in this picture, but it does no more than calculate. In fact, if I could get everything I wanted, I would not even have to calculate. I calculate, then, how I can get most of what I want or perhaps what I want most. I decide, for example, that I really want the Rolls Royce and therefore give up my vacation and my therapist. Or, I decide that I would rather have the vacation and keep seeing the therapist, and so give up the car. Individual desires are basic, and reason just enables me to do more efficiently what I already want to do.

Believers in individualism do know they need the services a society offers—police protection, for instance. But they only desire, and thus calculate about, those social matters that will help them get what they want. An individualist might not, then, see any reason to help the poor. This individualist position has had a very long history in the West, beginning in ancient Greece and continuing until present times. Many people, perhaps particularly Americans, accept it as the normal way to think about ethics.

The perfectionist position underlies most religious traditions in the West. Perfectionists assume there is a basis for judging whether human desires are good or bad, virtuous or vicious. They set standards—for example, that selfishness is bad and that compassion is good—and use those standards to judge themselves and others. Perfectionists do not simply start from the desires they have. Rather, they look to an ideal, a perfect human being, and try to act in a way that resembles such a person. The question they ask is not whether I can afford the Rolls Royce, but whether I ought to use that money to help the poor or to improve myself, say by studying meditation.

The ideal person who presents the standard is usually found in the dogma of a religious tradition—for example, in Jesus' willingness to sacrifice himself for the sake of other people. Perfectionists are guided not by humans *as they are* but by humans *as they can be* when they are most perfect. Reason does not calculate in this picture, but it does help people identify the standard of perfection and then move toward it. An important question that reason must deal with in the perfectionist picture is whether there is only one kind of perfect human state. For instance, can a person who is a great artist, but sacrifices little for the sake of others, be an appropriate ideal? Debate has raged around that issue in the West, but most traditions have claimed there is only one perfect state.

The rationalist position is most difficult to understand. It limits ethics to that small number of situations where we can say a universal rule applies. Reason, in this view, is defined as what allows people to recognize that a universal rule is applicable. Reason is crucial for two reasons. It alone can see universal rules. Moreover, it is only by understanding such rules that people can see why their individual desires ought not guide their actions. For example, suppose that I desire to mistreat a person simply because that person is a woman or a member of another religion. My reason will, or should, make me ask if I would make my desire a universal rule. Would I, for example, accept such mistreatment if it were directed at me? Presuming that I would reject the universality of such a rule, I then know I should not act that way and I overrule my desire. According to rationalism, reason discovers rules that apply universally, and only they should guide a person's ethical action.

Most Western governments rely on some version of rationalism when they consider the ethical rules that should guide everyone in a society. That is, rationalism guides governmental thinking about basic human rights, about the minimal conditions for any decent human life. It is a very influential position today. However, it is also a position with serious problems. Some proponents of rationalism go to the heart of the basic idea that making universal judgments should guide our actions. For example, one of the most famous philosophers in this tradition, Immanuel Kant, argues that no person ever should lie, because it is a universal reality that meaningful communication rests on the assumption that people tell the truth. However, suppose someone loans you a gun, and the person later returns in an agitated state, asking for the gun back because he wants to kill his sister. Kant would say you give the gun back because you ought not lie. Many have thought something is very wrong with a position that would lead to that decision.

Another, probably more important, problem arises from the fact that there seem to be few universal rules that reason can discover. This means ethics covers very little of what human life is about. That is, reason can show that no one should murder or steal, but after describing several such general rules, everything else a person does seems to depend only on the person's individual desires. This situation has meant that rationalism is often combined with individualism in the modern West. Many people follow a few strict universal rules defined by reason. However, in the rest of their lives, they are guided just by what they desire to do. Therefore, they use reason only to calculate how best to satisfy their desires.

One explanation as to why this combination is so prominent is that many people in the West reject perfectionism. Some do not accept the religious ideas on which it rests. Moreover, even if they accept such ideas, they think we cannot build a truly pluralistic society based on specific religious ideas, because some people hold different religious ideas or reject all religious ideas. Furthermore, many question perfectionist ideas because they think the West's history shows that people who hold such ideas have usually treated certain groups in terrible ways. Slavery, for example, and an inferior role for women were often justified by Christians.

Finally, perfectionism has also been rejected because it links human beings too closely to the rest of the natural world. Critics argue one cannot speak of the perfection of human nature in the same way one speaks of the perfection of a natural being. A beautiful oak tree is an example of a perfected oak seed, but there are too many different kinds of human perfection to say that only one of them is an example of a perfected human "seed." The operations of the natural world do not, then, provide an appropriate model for human perfection.

FOUR ARGUMENTS AGAINST COMPASSION AS THE BASIS OF AN ETHICAL SYSTEM

Although many Western religious traditions have stressed the importance of compassion, many modern Westerners believe compassion provides an insufficient basis for an ethical system—although all would agree that compassion is an important personal trait. These critics of compassion point to the fact that in spite of the ideal of compassion, Christianity and other traditions have tolerated many kinds of injustice. Most important, they believe that this fact is not simply a matter of chance, but shows the problems inherent in the idea of basing ethics on compassion. They argue that in addition to compassion, one needs the idea of rights—an idea that many think can only come from rationalism to establish a social situation in which all people are treated well.

For these critics, compassion rests on feelings that are unstable in all save the very best people. Most people normally feel compassion only at some times or toward some people. Therefore, the universal directives that only reason can give are needed. Moreover, they think compassion functions well only on a person-to-person level and therefore cannot produce the general guidelines we must have if we are to correct basic injustices in society. Compassion can tell me how to react to a suffering person I encounter on the street, but it alone cannot tell me what I should do to make sure that person, and others like that person, do not suffer any more.

Related to this is another criticism. Critics believe compassion almost always produces paternalism or, at least, problematic hierarchies—situations in which one group takes care of another group. This situation undermines the freedom of the people being cared for. That is, it reduces them to a childlike position and undercuts their ability to become fully free. For these critics of compassion, it is crucial that humans not be dependent, that they be able to choose freely—even if their choices are bad ones.

Compassion is also felt to be problematic because it is usually tied to a religious vision in which people's present life on earth is thought to be only a small part of the life they will live. Many critics believe these religious ideas about a life beyond one's present life either are untrue or at least are not proven in a scientifically valid way. Furthermore, they think it very important that humans recognize how little they know. Most critics also think these religious views lead virtually all people to be less concerned about the actual suffering they face than they otherwise would be. That is, people worry less about humanity's present suffering if their current plight is thought to be only a small part of their total life, a life that extends far beyond death in this world.

AN ETHICS WITHOUT RELIGION

DALAI LAMA: You spoke about the understanding of ethics from the Western point of view. My question is whether it is possible to formulate an ethical system without having to make any appeal to religious principles. Without accepting God or any mysterious forces, without accepting previous lives or karma, simply on the basis of the present life, is it possible to make some demarcation between virtue and nonvirtue, or to distinguish right from wrong?

LEE YEARLEY: Most modern ethics in the West has attempted to do exactly that. The rationalist position attempts to replace religious principles and still present acceptable reasons why people should not commit unethical behavior, at least in its most horrible forms. The crisis of ethics in the latter part of the twentieth century is that this position has left many kinds of action without any guidance whatsoever. You have these very general principles, but so much of what people do—how they treat their families, how they deal with minor theft, how they deal with their anger—seems not to be covered at all.

One response to this is the premise of Western ethics that society should be organized only on nonreligious principles, because there are too many religions and too many people who are not religious. A second, more challenging, idea is that the most critical thing for a human being is to choose freely whether or not to do something. They should never be guided by ideas that can't be scientifically proven, which includes religious ideas. If they make terrible mistakes, that's just the price human freedom exacts. Some of the best defenders of this liberal picture believe that, if the price of living without religious guidance is misspent lives, we just have to accept that and live with the results. At the deepest level, many of those who defend this system believe that one can know very little about anything. They argue that the best possible life is to recognize how little you can know about what a good life is.

D A L A I L A M A :   I think it's very important to try to present moral principles without any religious involvement. It is a reality now that out of five people, only one or two are religious believers. So, we must be seriously concerned with the remaining majority. Also, I sometimes feel it's easier to approach those nonbelievers. Compassion itself means something different in different ideologies. So a particular method of teaching compassion may not be acceptable to people who hold different beliefs. Even if the minds of nonbelievers are quite neutral about compassion, you must still find some way to reach those people. In Norway, I found a group of people who organized to promote human values, especially compassion, without any religious involvement.

COMPASSION AS A BASIS FOR ETHICS

S H A R O N   S A L Z B E R G :   Theravada Buddhism approaches ethics by distinguishing between what produces suffering and what ends suffering. This is even more exact than saying that actions are right or wrong, good or evil. This holds true both for oneself and for others. We cannot create suffering for ourselves without creating suffering for others, nor can we create suffering for others without creating suffering for ourselves. So the model of perfection for the highest development of the human being is someone who has come to the complete end of suffering himself or herself, and therefore will never create suffering for others. Therefore, it's absolutely essential that compassion is at the very foundation of the ethical system.

Also, when we use the word compassion, it doesn't carry the sense of a healthy person looking at a sick person. Maybe because we consider that we have all done so many different things over so many lifetimes, we don't think helping a person implies we are better than they are. We have been in their situation. So the compassion is a feeling of equality rather than that of a superior person looking at an inferior person.

The importance of compassion is also supported by the teaching that motivation is the most powerful and enduring part of an action. For example, if we give somebody something to eat because they are hungry, tomorrow they will be hungry again. Because of karma, the motive behind the action has a more powerful effect over a longer period of time than the action itself.[2]

DALAI LAMA: Various different religions all emphasize the importance of compassion. From the Buddhist viewpoint, I believe that compassion is an important aspect of human nature, part of the human mind. It is one of the good qualities of a human being. The various religions are trying to promote or strengthen that basic human quality, but this is not some external human acquisition, or some new invention by religious faith. It is already there, whether you are a Buddhist or not. There are so many various religions in existence, so religious practice is not necessarily the same as the practice of compassion. It is possible to present or promote loving kindness and compassion without religious connotation. Your point, Lee, was also well taken when you spoke of the inadequacy of compassion as the sole foundation of ethics, because if one has only altruism then this will be extremely limited, too limited. But compassion combined with wisdom and effective methods of service becomes something fuller, doesn't it?

JON KABAT-ZINN: Your Holiness, what is the perspective that wisdom brings that compassion alone does not afford?

DALAI LAMA: One application would be, to take Sharon's example, just alleviating another person's hunger for one day. If you applied wisdom, you would think further: How can I alter circumstances so this person doesn't suffer in the future or doesn't get into this predicament in the first place? Then again, when we talk about wisdom, there are different types. It means something different to a Buddhist or a non-Buddhist, for a start. Then, among Buddhists, there are many different kinds of wisdom.

I think non-Buddhists' wisdom is more practical; sometimes Buddhists' wisdom gets too sophisticated, too idealistic. The ideal is that all sentient beings should achieve Buddhahood through meditation practice. But to achieve that wisdom, it's not sufficient to show compassion or concern. You have to realize that unless people make an attempt to improve themselves, nothing can be done. It takes wisdom, not just sympathy, for people to move forward. But then, Buddhahood is too far off. [*laughter*]

LEE YEARLEY: People who argue that compassion is not enough say that even when linked with wisdom, it finally involves some people taking care of others. Compassion itself will never lead to the idea of human rights, for example, because that cannot be derived from a sympathetic understanding or loving kindness. It demands a whole different way of looking at the world. That's their argument, and I think it is historically correct that no matter how different traditions have emphasized compassion, they haven't usually coupled it with the idea of human rights, and terrible things have been done as a result.[3]

FRANCISCO VARELA: Is there no precedent in the West for what His Holiness was saying about not isolating compassion but combining it with a method—not necessarily wisdom—to elicit or bring about that compassion? Also, regarding perfectionism, you seem to always equate attaining the state of perfection with holding some kind of belief. But the belief need not be there. It could be an aspiration, with the method, without any particular heavy-handed set of theological beliefs.

LEE YEARLEY: There are parts of the main Western traditions, whether Jewish, Christian, or secular, that have used such methods, working with basic human impulses such as sympathy, and then training the self with methods like visualization. For example, one would think about the worst possible cases of lack of compassion and the best cases of compassion, read appropriate literature, and still the kinds of emotions that force one not to be compassionate.

FRANCISCO VARELA: But those cases are all bound to a belief. What about the early days of Marxism? There was an enormous aspiration for solidarity and compassion that was coupled with nonbelief in a religious system. There was some kind of method for building a society to fulfill these aspirations, although we know it wasn't particularly ideal how it ended.

LEE YEARLEY: I would say that Marxism, particularly in its early days, was about as powerful and fervent a religious movement as the West has seen in the last five hundred years. It had all the marks of a religion. Its justification lay far in the future. People were being asked to make tremendous self-sacrifices and train themselves for those self-sacrifices. It had very lofty goals, a founding figure who was revered, sacred texts that were studied. There was a very tight institution and tight organization of the people. It makes Roman Catholicism or Orthodox Judaism look rather meager.

Speaking for the critics of compassion, I think it is absolutely true that the great traditions where compassion is central, whether Buddhism, Christianity, or Confucianism, have always coexisted with societies where certain classes, such as women, peasants, or those without education, have been very deprived. No matter how universal the notion of compassion was, there was little or no drive or energy to improve the lot of these groups. Looking at what a religious basis for ethics has produced in the past, people have felt the need to start over again.

DANIEL BROWN: Lee, if I understand you correctly, compassion as a motivation for ethics in the West is criticized because it always involves inequality among people, some discrepancy in status or power or level of evolution. So, is inequality central to understanding this?

LEE YEARLEY: Inequality is central, but also important is the view of compassion assomething private, person to person.

DANIEL BROWN: Wouldn't the Buddhist practices that focus on the enlightenment of all beings, self and others, serve to avoid the problem of inequality in compassion?

DALAI LAMA: From the Buddhist viewpoint, there are different kinds and levels of compassion that vary with the individual practitioner and may reflect their other practices, such as wisdom or insight. In preliminary stages, compassion is usually mixed with desire or attachment. For example, the compassion between parent and child: you may have strong feelings of closeness and a sense of responsibility, but the reason is mainly a concern for something close to you. Because that kind of compassion is very much influenced by attachment, it's naturally very limited.

It's true that in specific circumstances where you have the ability to alleviate the suffering of another person or to protect another person from suffering, there is, in that sense, an inequality. One person has a capacity that the other person does not. But there is no such sense of inequality, no feeling of superiority, in the actual mode in which compassion views the other sentient being. It's absent. Compassion itself does not necessarily make the distinction between someone superior and someone below.

A deeper and broader type of compassion than one influenced by attachment is based mainly on a concern that the other being for whom I feel compassion is just like myself. That person wants happiness just like myself and has every right to be happy and to overcome suffering just like myself, whether that person is close to me or not. So long as they are a sentient being, particularly a human being with similar desires and rights, on *that* basis I develop compassion. That type of compassion is based on the equality of self and others. There's no room there for feeling superior. So actually *first* you realize that others have rights, and on that basis you develop the sense of concern and responsibility.

Ethics and Cultural Context

Daniel Goleman: If I could take Dr. Yearley's question one step further, he observed that historically many countries that were very religious, including Tibet, had peasant classes who lived in very bad conditions, and other classes who were very well off; and that the secular democratic rational approach to ethics would address this directly as an issue of human rights. How does it come about that such injustice exists along with such widespread teaching of compassion?

Dalai Lama: There's a simple thesis that people have "religion of the mouth"—they don't put their words into practice. However, I think if you compare the feudal system of Tibet with that of China or India, you see much more compassion and less suffering in the Tibetan system. Generally speaking, I believe the reason for this is the emphasis on compassion in the Buddha's teaching, but I would be interested to see research from less-biased people on this subject. Many foreigners have noticed that Tibetans are generally quite jovial and happy, on the face of it, especially those of the elder generation who were born and raised in the bad old system. Nobody says that Tibet in the past was perfect. Of course, there were a lot of negative defects and backwardness, but generally speaking it was quite a happy society. I think religion makes some differences. Before Buddhism flourished in Tibet, the Tibetans historically were a nation of warriors. Buddhism disqualified us for that. So, finally we lost our country. At the same time we have been able to create a lot of sympathizers.

When approaching the question of the proper foundation for ethical principles from a Buddhist point of view, you have to take into account the basic Buddhist notion of the interdependence of things. You can't say compassion is the only foundation; that if you have that, everything will be perfect and if you do not have that, nothing will be perfect. Compassion can be a motive for ethical actions, but that doesn't mean compassion alone is sufficient. From a Buddhist viewpoint, all three positions of Western ethics that Dr. Yearley mentioned—individualism, rationalism, and perfectionism—have valid grounds for their theses.

Individualism is valid in that every individual must work for his or her own benefit, his or her own fulfillment, and you have to take into account a person's individual desires. Similarly, you have to also take perfectionism into account, because what we are aiming for is a perfect state of existence. Thirdly, you have to take into account rationalism, because we need the human rational faculty to make judgments about what is right and what is wrong in a particular context. So, from the Buddhist point of view you cannot say any one thing is the foundation of ethics; you have to take into account their interdependent nature. Each of those three is necessary, but none of the three will adequately stand alone. Likewise, compassion alone is not an adequate basis for ethics, but that doesn't mean compassion is not the right motive or foundation for ethics.

LEE YEARLEY: In Western ethics, those three ideas cannot be brought together at all, or at least not very easily, because when you say individual desires are important, you either mean that anything any individual wants is all right, or that some desires are better than other desires. Once you begin to distinguish good desires from bad ones, you are really a perfectionist. In the West, the individualist position maintains that the individual is the only important thing in the whole universe: whatever that individualist wants, he or she should attempt to get it, and the state should allow him or her to have it. If you are looking for a religious principle in modern Western ethics, that's probably it. It's not very clear that it makes much sense except as a religious principle. The rationalist position is a very good example of how much some people can treasure their own particular view of rationality, because it depends on the possibility of convincing people not to do things simply because they are wrong.

DALAI LAMA: Given this rationalist position, there might be certain acts for which we have a consensus regarding right or wrong, but in many cases the judgment depends on a specific context. You have to take into account the different circumstances, the people that were involved, their mental dispositions, and so forth. Therefore, how do the rationalists account for the fact that an act may be justified for one individual, but may not be suitable for another person?

LEE YEARLEY: In Western terms, His Holiness is presenting a very good position in the tradition of Aristotle or Thomas Aquinas. But a rationalist would claim the situation makes absolutely no difference. Remember, Kant argued that no person should ever lie, because meaningful communication is based on the assumption of truth. Think about my example about the person loaning you a gun and later asking for it back because he wants to kill his sister. Kant would say you give the gun back, because you cannot lie. As you have said, and others would agree, it is not right that this philosophical position would condone this outcome.

DALAI LAMA: This example shows the relativity of the very concept of what is right and what is wrong. So, ultimately, decisions should be made on the basis of what is beneficial and what is harmful. It's consequences that determine whether an action is right or wrong. Any action that leads to a harmful consequence can be judged wrong, and an action that leads to beneficial consequences can be considered as a right action.

LEE YEARLEY: This leads to another problem that comes up in this tradition. If you think only in terms of bene-

fits and consequences, you also seem to find some very difficult cases.

DALAI LAMA: That's why motivation and compassion
are important.

FRANCISCO VARELA: In this view of perfectionism
that you see as a possibility, do you see some pragmatics or
method as an integral part of it, and if so what kind? I ask
the question because it seems to me, as a Westerner raised in
a Christian context, completely absent from the perfectionist
view, that, for example, you are told to love, but you fail
miserably when you try.

LEE YEARLEY: I think this is one place where actually
there are wonderful riches in the Western traditions. They
don't just tell you to be compassionate, be loving, but instead
give you practices or exercises to do. But many people hold
this picture that they are only told what one ought to be,
and then fail miserably, and therefore decide that the Western
traditions are somehow bankrupt. It just shows how much
the tradition has lost touch with its own roots and absorbed
certain very questionable aspects of the modern world. One
of these is the notion that if you understand something, you
will somehow immediately be able do it. I think this comes
as one result of the rationalist picture that the thought itself
leads naturally and normally to the action. None of the
deeper parts of the Western tradition, in Judaism, Christianity, or anywhere else, ever thought that was true.

DALAI LAMA: So your conclusion is that in order to
have a consistent ethical principle, we are forced to make appeal to religious or transcendental ideas that cannot scientifically be proven? When you say you endorse a perfectionist
model, does this mean that you really do need to resort to
some sort of religion to establish that ethical basis?

LEE YEARLEY: Yes, most emphatically. I think you
have to use religious practices and religious ideas, and I think
you have to draw on energies or powers that are not part of
the normal human experience.

DALAI LAMA: What about animals, especially social animals? They have a limited form of altruism and it also seems they have a very good sense of responsibility to the common benefit, but without any religion.

LEE YEARLEY: There are surely resources that humans have naturally that you can draw on to help them build community and meet obligations. I am much saddened by the history of the West because people seem to be less and less able to operate ethically without religious grounding. Often people could act responsibly in the past even when they were not religious because they were drawing in some way on a culture or a tradition that was religious. It seems that part of the reason America is in such desperate trouble now is that people are completely removed from a religious basis. They are told they have to belong to a country, contribute to it, and meet basic rights, but they don't, and there is almost no way to convince them or to make them.

DALAI LAMA: Do you believe that ethical principles of right and wrong are relative to a particular religious community, or are you saying there are some universal truths which all human beings share?

LEE YEARLEY: The last twenty years of my life have been spent trying to deal with that question. I think there are some remarkable similarities, at least among the religions or cultures I know something about, and I find that uplifting. But speaking about those truths seems to require a language that goes beyond what a particular tradition offers. Neither a Confucian nor a Christian nor a Buddhist way of talking about these things is fully adequate. We need a new way of talking about them without completely losing touch with the traditions of which we are a part. It seems to me finding that new language is absolutely critical.

THUBTEN JINPA: So you're saying there are universally shared religious truths that can be put in the context of different religious languages?

LEE YEARLEY: That's what I'm saying right now. I have been a long time reaching that position and I am not sure what position I will be in five years from now.

A UNIVERSAL BASIS FOR ETHICS

FRANCISCO VARELA: His Holiness's question about social animals manifesting a very responsible altruism simply out of compassion, with of course no religious or cultural context, implies that the mainspring of such values may not necessarily be religious tradition. Not that it couldn't be, but why should that be the only one?

LEE YEARLEY: This is a point on which there is dispute, but one ethical position has argued that what is so distinctive about human beings is that they are not as easily communal as other animals; that what is most unique and perhaps worthwhile about us is also what is most potentially horrible: that we don't necessarily sacrifice for the group, we don't necessarily love those who are close to us. We can decide simply to pursue our own very clever ways, and be successful. I think humans and animals are just radically different, at least on that particular ground, but I know there are many scientists who also consider themselves ethicists who would disagree.

FRANCISCO VARELA: That's why I'd like to go into this question, because I am a biologist.

DALAI LAMA: That freedom of choice can be our greatest strength, but it can also be our greatest detriment.

FRANCISCO VARELA: His Holiness was suggesting there might be some basic capacity that is not particularly religious, but could be used as grounds for ethics. Returning to the question about animals, I've always felt that in animals the natural compassion for their kind has a very fuzzy edge. We know of examples of compassion that are intraspecific—between species. The symbol of Rome is two children,

Romulus and Remus, who were fed by a wolf. That she-wolf wasn't acting for her species. There was something intrinsically there that allowed her to overstep the boundary between species and to feed human children.

LEE YEARLEY: But that is a religious symbol. It has meaning precisely because it is not biologically based, and that's why the Romans took it as their symbol.

FRANCISCO VARELA: However, it does happen, biologically. There are many reports of dolphins helping sailors.

LEE YEARLEY: There's no question it happens biologically, but I think humans took it on precisely because of the oddness.

FRANCISCO VARELA: But if there's something there that doesn't start with culture, that is an enormous base on which to build, a base you can expand by training.

DALAI LAMA: In terms of human development, isn't it the case that this occurs in the relationship between parent and child or between the sexes? That's why the human population grows and grows. Even in plants, there is some kind of cooperation. Human society is based on the human family, and the family is based on cooperation, not by force but by necessity. The initial necessity then produces a positive result, a satisfaction, and so the family grows. So this happens on the basis of the positive qualities of human nature. Religion does not come into it yet; this is a basic quality of the human mind. Of course, anger and jealousy are also produced from our mind. However, I think the dominant force of our mind is human compassion and affection. If the dominant force were anger, then family could not develop. Killing and bullying people doesn't produce a family, but humanity does exist. Now, we are worried about overpopulation as a result. Human nature is basically positive: that is the basis of religion from the Buddhist point of view. Anyway, religion is humankind's creation. Of course, it's possible to see God as something external to humankind, but even if there is a God, if there is no human being, no receiver, you cannot develop religion. The main contribution comes from human beings. So religion is based on the good qualities of human nature, on intrinsic affection. When people realize something good there, something of benefit, then they try to strengthen that quality and enforce it. Of course, on certain occasions it may be allowable to express anger. However, no religion encourages anger as something beneficial, because anger creates problems. Human beings do not appreciate anger; they don't like destruction. I think rather they love construction.

LEE YEARLEY: Why do they destroy so much, then?

DALAI LAMA: If we look at history over all the millions of years that human beings have existed, I think there has been more construction than destruction. Ordinarily, when something destructive happens we are shocked, because by nature we are affectionate and gentle. When nice things happen, we take them for granted. Destruction makes a bigger impression, so we think there is more destruction than something gentler like construction. Can you argue this further? I've always thought it very important to hear a different viewpoint.

LEE YEARLEY: I remain drawn to, if not convinced by, what seems to me the deepest strain inside the Christian tradition, which holds that everything you've said about human beings is correct—they construct, they build families—but that there is also something inside humans that moves toward destruction, violation, and self-hurt, something that is obscured and finds itself in darkness, that has tendencies to strike out even at things it once loved. It is inexplicable but it exists, and the whole Christian tradition is trying to deal with the question of why there is this deep evil inside people, in spite of everything you've said. As one Christian theologian put it, original sin shouldn't be but clearly is.

DANIEL GOLEMAN: Is there a Buddhist equivalent of original sin or evil?

DALAI LAMA: The Buddhist equivalent would be fundamental ignorance.

JON KABAT-ZINN: That's a very compassionate view of evil, to call it ignorance. Lee, you have painted a very fine picture of a serious dilemma, an epistemological problem. What is your personal view of whether resolution is possible here?

LEE YEARLEY: I have convinced myself, and a few friends, that resolution is possible. I think it rests on a perfectionist picture of people. I also think part of what that means is you're never going to be able to convince some people about the rightness of this picture, which is distressing in some ways.

JON KABAT-ZINN: But how would this picture look different from the earlier perfectionist picture with its dilemmas?

LEE YEARLEY: I think some aspects of the rationalist picture, including notions of rights and justice, can be introduced into the perfectionist picture. I have more trouble with how you attempt to bring a perfectionist picture into existence in a free democratic society. That seems to me controlling people in ways that are very problematic.

JON KABAT-ZINN: Do you think that science, or the broader perspective on the mind/body connection, holds any promise of making a contribution to this new perfectionist picture that would make it substantially different from earlier perfectionist cul-de-sacs?

DANIEL GOLEMAN: In other words, do we have the basis for a new morality?

LEE YEARLEY: I have my doubts, but maybe I'll be convinced.

NOTES

1. The labels used for each of these ethical positions differ from those used in technical discussions in the West.

2. The Buddhist concept of karma is a process of cause and effect

in which motives and actions produce physical and mental effects for the person who has engaged in the actions, as well as for the recipients of the actions. For example, a man who gives food to another, because of his compassion, has increased his tendency to engage in altruistic behavior.

3. The "whole different way of looking at the world" that leads to the concept of human rights evolves from the rationalist view of ethics. According to the rationalist point of view, for example, the concept of human rights is an abstract one. It does not depend on particular sentiments, but on general logical principles. The fundamental principle of the metaphysic of morals, according to Immanuel Kant, asserts that one must act "as if the maxim from which you act were to become through your will a universal law." When this principle is applied to human relations, it logically obliges one to treat others not merely as means to an end, but as ends in themselves. Others intrinsically have rights. Other Western philosophers, such as the empiricist John Locke, believed that humans had rights. In Locke's view, there was natural law, which preceded organized society. According to Locke, the natural state was a happy one characterized by reason and tolerance. He believed that humans had the right to pursue life, liberty, and property.

2

Afflictive and Nourishing Emotions: Impacts on Health

DANIEL GOLEMAN

O UR EMOTIONS can matter greatly to our health. On one hand, the weight of scientific data shows that the link between emotions and health is particularly strong for negative feelings: anger, anxiety, and depression. These states, if strong and prolonged, can increase vulnerability to disease, worsen the symptoms, or hinder recovery. On the other hand, more positive states like equanimity and optimism seem to have salutary effects on health— although the data on the health impact of positive emotions is not as strong as for negative ones. Daniel Goleman reviews the evidence and the possible implications of using biological imperatives for health as a guideline for ethical action.

DANIEL GOLEMAN: Your Holiness, you raised the point that 3 to 4 billion people on the planet have no religious belief. The question is, what kind of ethics can appeal to those 4 billion? I'm going to present experimental scientific evidence suggesting a completely new path for approaching that question: that the body's own mind, the immune system, provides a basis for a de facto ethical system in the difference between emotional states that help one stay healthy and live longer, and those that promote disease. What I'm going to show is that the body's ethical system, this "body dharma," approximates an aspect of Buddhadharma, in that the afflictive emotions tend to make one ill and wholesome states of mind tend to promote health. In looking at the new scientific evidence, I am struck by how similar the states of mind that lead to illness or to health are to those described as those that are wholesome or unwholesome in many ancient spiritual systems like Buddhism or Christianity.

Let me first give a context for the research I'll be talking about. In looking at the states of mind that lead to being well or ill, I don't want to imply that the mental states are all that's involved. When you consider why we get sick at any given time, there are many factors. We are constantly exposed to germs or cells in the body starting to become tumors, and although the immune system is continually patrolling for these, there are many things that can weaken it. One is heredity: we can inherit a genetic tendency to autoimmune disease, to cancer, or to other specific diseases. Another factor is bad habits: smoking leads to lung disease; not eating properly weakens the immune system. Environment is also a factor: air pollution in modern times has caused a great increase in breathing problems such as asthma.

The new discovery in the last five or ten years is that states of mind can affect the strength of the immune system and the robustness of the cardiovascular system. The particular emotional states I'm going to review are the only ones on which there has so far been scientific research to any degree. The afflictive states reviewed are anger or hostility; depression, which includes not just sadness, but also self-pity, guilt, and hopelessness; stress, which covers agitation, nervousness, and anxiety; and repression, or the denial of anxiety. The beneficial states reviewed are calm, optimism, confidence, joy, and loving kindness.

The impact of these states on the immune system is measured by the increase or decrease in the number of immune cells or in their effectiveness. The prevailing view in the medical profession has been that the range of immune-cell shifts with emotion documented so far does not have a great impact on health, but that may change with the new evidence. To put this range of immune shifts in perspective: if, for instance, you weaken the immune system of white rats by applying repeated electric shocks, when their immune capacity is reduced by about 80 percent, the rats start to die of different illnesses because their immune effectiveness is severely impaired. But that does not happen with a drop of 20 to 30 percent—the range found in most studies of emotions and immune function—although one can argue that this range of change still seems to make a difference in how well you fight the germs that come your way and how soon you recover from sickness. And the research on these states of mind also includes heart disease and other diseases that don't have anything to do with the immune system, so they seem to affect health in general.

The whole idea that states of mind can affect health at all is very new in science, and it's telling what states have not been studied. For instance, there are no studies of the effect of greed on health, because greed is not considered a problem or a pathology in the West; it's a cultural norm. And while looking at different qualities of mind in meditation and how they affect different diseases is a promising idea, it's way beyond where science is right now. But there is a large body of data about ordinary emotions and health.

The first state of mind is anger. Dr. John Barefoot at the University of North Carolina tested people who had symptoms of potentially serious heart disease. When they came in for a procedure to measure blockage in the arteries, they were given a psychological test to see how angry they were in general. They were asked, for instance, how often they yelled at their children. The lowest amount of blockage was found in the group that had the least anger, and the people that had the most anger had the highest blockage. Now this doesn't prove that anger blocks the arteries, because some third factor may cause both the anger and the blockage.

So we look for a prospective study, which predicts how a

person will be in the future based on how they are now. Dr. Redford Williams at Duke University looked at a group of 2,000 factory workers who happened to have taken a test about twenty-five years earlier that included a measure of their level of hostility. Of those who had a very low score for anger, up to 20 percent had died. About 30 percent of those with a high level of anger had died, from causes such as heart disease, cancer, other diseases, and from causes not even related to health, such as accidents. This suggests that if you're a chronically angry person, you're one and a half times more likely to die, over a period of twenty-five years, than a person who's not angry.

We would presume that the accidents among these people were caused by anger, but we don't know for sure. Since then other studies have shown that anger is an even stronger factor in early death. In one study begun in the mid-1950s, a group of medical students were tested and classified as chronically hostile or not. When Williams tracked them down twenty years later, only 3 of the 136 who were not rated as highly hostile had died. Sixteen of the group with greater hostility had died, so it's a factor that seems to greatly heighten the risk of death. The interesting thing is that most of the deaths among those who were angry happened before age fifty: the angry seem to die young.

Dr. Williams has also carefully studied the particular quality of anger that seems to lead to early death, and found that it has three parts. First is the attitude of cynicism. If you have a suspicious, negative view of people, you assume they are probably going to threaten you so you had better be on guard. This constant attitude of hostility then leads to the feeling of anger, and the feeling in turn leads to action: having outbursts of anger, yelling at people, complaining impatiently.

Researchers at Harvard Medical School found that the single emotion most common in the two hours prior to a serious heart attack was anger. Once heart disease develops, anger appears particularly lethal. In people who have already had one heart attack, a bout of rage can lower the pumping efficiency of the heart by 7 percent or more, a range cardiologists regard as a dangerous drop in blood flow to the heart. And in studies at Stanford and at Yale medical schools, those people who had suffered a first heart attack and were most easily roused to anger were two to three times more likely than other patients to die of a later heart attack over the next decade.

The risk from hostility may be greater for men than for women. Testosterone is the hormone that, during development in the womb, makes the baby become a male. Men have much more of it than women do. This hormone may heighten aggressiveness, although there is a debate on the question. But people who commit violent crimes tend to have higher-than-usual levels of testosterone. If you have a high level of testosterone, you like to control situations, and so you tend to be argumentative or fight more often. It seems to make you more vulnerable to heart disease.

The next state of mind with adverse health consequences is depression: feeling sadness, self-pity, or hopelessness. There are many studies, which I'll just cover briefly. The weight of evidence for depression is stronger for interfering with recovery from severe illness than as an initial cause of disease. For example, in a study of women with breast cancer, the most depressed women had the fewest natural killer cells. It's believed that part of the job of these cells is to fight cancer by patrolling the body for tumors starting to grow. The depressed patients had the fewest of these cells, and also had tumors spreading more quickly to different parts of the body.

At Mt. Sinai Medical School in New York City, psychiatrists evaluated levels of depression in elderly people who came to the hospital with a broken hip—a very serious injury, since they may never walk again. Those who were not depressed were three times more likely than those who were depressed to walk again, and nine times more likely to return to their previous level of health. So the depression seemed to interfere with healing the bone, or with recovering function.

At the University of Minnesota, of 100 patients who received bone marrow transplants, 12 of the 13 who before the surgery had been seriously depressed died within the first year of the transplant, while 34 of the remaining 87 were alive two years later. Depression also poses a medical risk for heart attack survivors. At the University of Montreal, among patients treated for a first heart attack, the one in eight who were seriously depressed afterward were five times more likely to die than were patients with comparable heart disease but no depression.

Let's move on to anxiety, or stress, which is called agitation or restlessness in the Abhidharma system. In one experiment they caged five male monkeys who had never seen each other before. Monkeys by nature like to have a commander in chief. They determine who is the boss by fighting with each other; once they decide, everybody else follows orders and everything is peaceful. Every month the researchers took out two monkeys and put in two new monkeys, which meant the monkeys had to fight all over again to establish the hierarchy. They did this for a year and also kept a separate group of five monkeys without change. After a year they found that the monkeys who were changed had blocked arteries. The boss monkey had the worst heart disease because he was the one fighting the most. It's interesting that the boss monkey in the other group had the least blockage—it's healthier to be the boss if no one's fighting.

Another way of looking at anxiety was a study of people who lived near the nuclear reactor at Three Mile Island. Blood samples from those who lived near the reactor and were therefore anxious and apprehensive had fewer T-cells and B-cells than samples taken from people in a similar neighborhood distant from the nuclear plant. So fear and worry seem to have an impact on the immune system.

But studies of immune changes are more ambiguous than those that also show a related illness effect. For example, at Ohio State University medical students studying for their major exams, and so under great stress, had large drops in T-cell and B-cell levels, as well as a higher number of colds and flus.

The best data has come from work at a special colds research unit in England, in association with researchers at Carnegie-Mellon University, who systematically expose volunteers to cold viruses. Not everyone so exposed gets a cold—it depends on the robustness of their immune system at the time. But here stress and anxiety seem crucial. Of people undergoing little stress at the time they were exposed to the cold virus, 27 percent came down with a cold; of those undergoing high stress, 47 percent got a cold.

Finally, the overall picture seems to suggest that all agitating, distressing states of mind heighten health risks. Howard Friedman, at the University of California at Irvine, analyzed data from over 100 studies linking people's predominant emotional states to their health. When compared to average people, those who tended to be unusually hostile and angry, very anxious, sad, pessimistic, or tense, had double the risk of getting a serious illness, including asthma, chronic headaches, stomach ulcers, heart disease, and arthritis.

The final afflictive emotion that has had much research is repression or denial. I believe this is, in a general sense, related to aspects of ignorance or delusion in the Abhidharma. Gary Schwartz and colleagues then at Harvard did research some years ago on the facial muscles that express emotion, particularly the muscle at the center of the forehead, which tenses when you're worried. People who get many headaches often have a high tension level in this muscle. Sometimes the muscle is tense without showing a wrinkle, so they use an electrode to detect the tension. Some people who had high muscle tension said they felt fine and were not worried. When they studied these people further, they found that they were denying what actually was going on in their body. The researchers would do things to agitate them physically, measure their muscle tension and heart rate, which are signs of physical agitation, and then ask them whether they felt relaxed or tense. Most people say they are tense when their bodies are tense, but these people claimed *not* to be tense when their bodies were. These people are said to be in denial.

People who are "repressors" like this may be more susceptible to diseases like asthma, high blood pressure, and colds.

Women with breast cancer who are repressors may be more likely to have a return of the tumor. So again, repression seems to be bad for health.

WHOLESOME EMOTIONS AND HEALTH

Looking at wholesome mental states, we see just the opposite picture. Consider equanimity, or a state of calm. Most of the studies have been done on people who learn some way to relax, very often meditation. They find these calming practices really relax the body—what Dr. Herbert Benson at Harvard University calls the relaxation response—and there are many, many health benefits.

There are a range of methods used clinically to help people become more calm. In biofeedback, for instance, an electrode on the muscle at the center of the forehead of people who tend to worry helps them hear a sound from the machine every time this muscle tenses, and so learn to prevent the sound by relaxing. They learn to relax more effectively, because now they can identify when the muscle is tense or relaxed. This state of calm has many health benefits. I pointed out that T-cells and B-cells decrease in students taking exams. When some of the students at Ohio State University who were facing exams meditated every day, their T-cells were found to increase instead. The more often and more consistently they meditated, the stronger the effect.

Optimism, the next positive state of mind, is really more an outlook, a view that has to do with how you explain the bad things that happen in your life, which in turn can keep you from becoming depressed or demoralized in the face of setbacks. In failing an exam, for example, some people would say they failed because they are stupid. They explain it in terms of some fixed, permanent trait in themselves. That's the negative or pessimistic view. Others would say they failed because it was a very hard test, but next time they'll study harder. They explain bad things happening in terms of a constantly changing situation—a more Buddhist view, I think. They are hopeful that things will be different next time. In one study started in the 1940s, students at Harvard University were classified as pessimists or optimists based on essays they had written explaining events in their lives. About thirty years later, the health history of these same students after leaving school was examined. Starting in their forties, the pessimists had more serious diseases and health problems than the optimists. At the University of Michigan, similar classification was made of people undergoing bypass surgery; the optimists had fewer problems during the surgery and made a faster recovery. So even in that intense situation, optimism seemed to be good for health.

Another positive state of mind is confidence, a sense of being able to handle the situation. In the West it's often thought of as a sense of control. A confident person feels things are in their control. Certain jobs make people feel they have little control. For instance, a bus driver is supposed to keep a certain schedule. He's expected to be there no matter what happens, but all kinds of things can happen on the way that he can't control. People in such jobs have about three times as much high blood pressure and other medical problems compared to those in jobs where they have more control over what they do.

In one experiment repeated at several medical centers, two white rats are put in cages next to each other. Both rats get an electric shock simultaneously, but one rat has a lever it can push to stop the shock, and the other has no lever. They get exactly the same shock, but only one can control it. The one without control gets stomach ulcers. When both rats are injected with cancer cells, the tumors spread more rapidly in the rat without control.

People in nursing homes often feel they have no control, especially as many nursing homes are run very strictly. Yale psychologists convinced the people running one nursing home to let a group of elderly people have more control over decisions such as what they would eat or when they would have visitors; they also gave each individual in this group a plant to take care of. A year later, the group had half as many deaths as others who had no sense of control.

Another very important state of mind is friendliness, or in psychological terms, social connection— the extent to which an individual has many friends, or people providing emotional support. Again, researchers looked at students taking exams, which is a natural experiment for stress. Those who felt most lonely had the fewest natural killer cells during exams. In women with breast cancer, those who had the most social support had 30 percent more natural killer cells than women without such connections.

In a study at the University of California, researchers interviewed 5,000 people house to house in a big city and looked at how many friends they had, how many people who cared about them. This included not just having friends but various ways that people participated in their community: in civic organizations, in church, at public meetings, at local school meetings for their children—the sense of connection to the wider community. After nine years, the people who had very few friends were twice as likely to have died as those who had very many. Many other studies have found this factor of social contact connected to death rates.

Because of a series of findings like this showing that human connections buffer the effects of stress, people who are ill are increasingly placed in groups for emotional support with others who have the same disease. This was a very controversial idea, that having people who care about you and caring about other people could help your health. About ten years ago, Dr. David Spiegel at Stanford University tried this with women who had advanced cases of breast cancer, on the assumption that it couldn't hurt and it might help them cope emotionally with what at that point was an almost certainly fatal disease. One group was given the usual medical treatment. The other group had the usual medical treatment but also met for group therapy once a week for a year. They talked about their feelings concerning the cancer and what it meant for their families. They became very close as a group, with a lot of love being generated in these meetings. They also learned a self-hypnosis technique for pain control.

The researchers then studied the death rate of both groups over the next ten years. After two or three years, the groups started to show differences. The women who had participated in group therapy died less rapidly than those who got only the regular medical treatment. After ten years, the death rate was twice as great in the group that only had medical treatment.

This has also been studied in animals. A caged monkey was subjected to flashing bright lights and loud banging sounds, and then the hormone cortisol, which the body releases in response to stress or fear and which also suppresses the immune system, was measured. When another monkey was placed in the same cage, only half as much of the hormone was released. With five other monkeys in the cage, the lights and noises had no effect at all on the level of cortisol secreted.

In a similar case, rabbits were being studied for heart disease. They were fed very rich foods that block the arteries. Some of the rabbits were picked up and petted affectionately. The rabbits that were petted had less blockage than those that were not petted.

Another positive mental state is joy, or happiness. Harvard researchers measured the hormones of people watching funny movies and found that the level of cortisol was reduced and the number of natural killer cells increased. So laughing matters, although we can't say if it has a medically significant effect. Another study found that watching funny movies increased the number of T-cells, and people who laughed a lot in everyday life showed the biggest increase in T-cells during the film. A similar study looked at thirty-six women with breast cancer who had had tumors. Some of the women had no further problem, but in others the cancer recurred. After seven years, twenty-four of the women had died. Earlier psychological tests showed that the only emotional difference between the ones who survived and the ones who died was a sense of joy in life. The researchers were very surprised that joy turned out to be a more powerful predictor of who would

die and who would live than how many sites the cancer had
spread to. (This data needs to be replicated before any strong
conclusions can be drawn.)

Finally, loving kindness—although the data here is scanti-
est and most speculative. Dr. David McClelland at Harvard
had some people watch a very loving film about Mother Teresa caring for people. Others watched a movie about the
Nazis in Germany, which made them very angry. There was
a brief rise in the number of T-cells in those who watched the
film about Mother Teresa. If, after watching the film, they
also spent an hour in loving kindness meditation, thinking
about all the people in their lives who'd been very kind to
them, the rise in T-cells lasted longer. Inducing this state of
mind seemed to bring out and strengthen the T-cells and the
immune system generally—although we don't know that the
range of change in immune functions here has any real medical significance.

Those are the main studies so far, both on negative and
positive states of mind. It seems there is very clear, strong
evidence for their effect on health—especially the deleterious
impact of strong, chronic negative emotions. This area of
medical research is very new, and many of these clinical studies have to be repeated several times to be sure that the effects
are real and robust. And for those studies that rely on immune measures, we do not yet know if there is any real medical impact from the range of changes observed in most of
them—they are merely suggestive, not definitive. The strongest data come from studies that have used disease or death
as an outcome measure, and even here the more often other
researchers confirm the findings, the surer we can be of these
links between emotions and health.

Still, if these scientific trends continue to be verified by future findings, this might provide an answer to the problem
that Lee talked about: how to convince people to live ethically who have no religious belief but only the individualistic
ethic, "Whatever I want is what I should get." Perhaps you
can say it's in their self-interest to be loving, not to be angry.

DALAI LAMA: You've given me a lot of ammunition! (*laughter*)

CAVEATS

FRANCISCO VARELA: A comment about the biology of the evidence that Dan has talked about. The measurements reflect global parameters and activity on a very general, unspecific scale. It's like taking your temperature: it can tell you something general about the state of your body, but the fever might be caused by one of thirty different things. A measurement of amounts of T-cells is similarly a very rough global parameter that could mean many things in terms of the relative activity of different key aspects of the system. And taking an EEG is like putting a microphone in the middle of a city. You may be able to distinguish whether the city is quiet or not, but you cannot infer the exchange rate of dollars to francs from that. The immune system, like the brain, is very specific. The suppression or elevation of T-cells is a very large, blurry measurement that cannot tell you, for example, whether a factor is more favorable to healing wounds or preventing cancer.

So we touch here on techniques that are just starting to develop, and we have to be content with very gross measurements that might be misleading. We have to be very, very prudent in not being overly optimistic in interpreting these kinds of initial studies.

DANIEL BROWN: Some of the better studies do go one step further, in that they not only measure changes in global immune functioning such as T-cell numbers but also measure variations in the incidence of illness. For example, in the study on the medical students, as well as measuring immune function, you can also develop correlations between the immune activity and the incidence of illness. Researchers were able to show that when the immune measures went down, the people got more illnesses. Studies of mortality are also a very concrete measure that these things have a negative or a positive effect. But an increase in the number of natural killer cells is a very rough indicator. The cytotoxicity percentage is a better measure of the natural killer cells' efficiency, because it shows that the cells are doing something to defend against disease rather than just how many there are.

FRANCISCO VARELA: Another example of more specific measures: In myasthenia gravis, we were able to measure increases or decreases of five particular clones [for antibodies] that are known to be very relevant to this disease. The approach is fine-tuned rather than global, like putting a small electrode inside the brain and measuring specific cell activity. This kind of study is much more meaningful, but it's much harder to do.

PART TWO

==

Biological Foundations

3

The Body's Self

FRANCISCO VARELA

FRANCISCO VARELA, in describing the structure and function of the immune system, calls it "the second brain." He makes an analogy between the immune system and the nervous system, pointing out that both are self-regulating and control the responses of the body to the environment. The immune system, like the nervous system, can remember, learn, and so adapt, not in a cognitive sense, but in a physiological one. The interaction between the mind, the nervous system, and the immune system provides a physiological basis for the influence of emotions on health. Evidence for the strength of this interaction include that stress experienced by the nervous system hampers the functioning of the immune system, and that immune responses can be conditioned like Pavlov's dogs learning to salivate at the sound of a bell. The study of this responsive attuning between the nervous system and the immune system is called psychoneuroimmunology (*psyche* for mind, *neuro* for nervous system, and for the immune system, *immunology*), a new subfield of biology. The premise of interdependence between neurology, immunology, and psychology forms a conceptual basis for much of the ensuing explorations in this book.

FRANCISO VARELA: My research is concerned with the biological bases of knowledge in all its forms, and I will be describing the immune system within this context. Psychoneuroimmunology is the study of the relationships between the nervous system, the immune system, and states of mind. This is a new field in the West, not more than fifteen years old, and an exciting one because it engenders an understanding of the mind/body connection.

When you ask how emotions affect the body, you need to consider the nervous system and how the brain works, and to realize that the immune system functions as a second brain of the body—not just metaphorically but concretely.

THE BODY'S SECOND BRAIN

The first question we ask about a system is: What is its organ? Like the components of the nervous system, the organs of the immune system are dispersed throughout the body. They include the thymus and bone marrow, the sources from which the system is constantly renewed; the spleen; and the lymphatic system, a network of tissue nodes connected by conduits through which the lymph fluid circulates.

The cells that constitute the immune system are called lymphocytes, or white blood cells, and are circulating all the time, unlike the fixed neurons of the nervous system. Most lymphocytes are produced in the bone marrow and therefore are called B-cells. Thymal cells, or T-cells, are produced in the thymus. Although fewer in number, the T-cells control the B-cells, like officers regulating soldiers.

The cells of the nervous system are distinguished by their shape and location. For instance, the neurons in the visual cortex are distinct from those in the hippocampus. Lymphocytes are not identified by location, since they circulate, but by their *cell receptors*. These are macromolecules on the cell's surface that interact with the receptors of other cells as they circulate. The cell receptors are markers that enable us to identify a cell's specific function, much as we can recognize a specific neuron in the brain.

Among these markers are the macromolecules called antibodies. B-cells are identified by unique *antibodies*, shared by as few as twenty or thirty other cells in the immune system. They are little families of B-cell clones producing identical antibodies that are markers, like a unique family name. In a normal immune system, there are about a 100 million different clone families circulating, each distinguishable by its unique antibodies. Imagine a large city of 100 million families, each with specific affinities to others, and all of them moving around. It's quite complex.

Like other receptors on the surface of the cells, antibodies have a very specific shape that can bind with any of a variety of molecules whose shapes are complementary. As an analogy, if I cup my hand slightly, an apple or an orange would be able to enter that space and bind for a moment, but the same hand position would not be a good fit for a pen. A B-cell binds very quickly with any cell or bacterium, or anything floating in the blood with the specific molecular shape that fits. There is a very rapid exchange, back and forth, binding and unbinding. These interactions are a method of communication, just as neurons communicate by sending electrical impulses.

In the nervous system, the most important events are the activation and inhibition of neurons. Most of neuroscientific analysis focuses on measuring this relative amount of activity. There is an exact analogy in the activation or suppression of B-cells and T-cells in the immune system. Here, activation refers to the cells dividing so that the clone family increases in number. Suppression means a decrease in the number of clones as the cells die off.

The normal life span of a B-cell in a human is between one and two days, although some live slightly longer. This means that the system is renovated very rapidly on a vast scale. After a week or two, the lymphocytes have all been replaced. What remains, therefore, is a *pattern*: the kinds of clones and their degree of activation. This, of course, is unlike the brain, where by and large the neurons neither die nor reproduce.

There are still other important analogies between the nervous system and the immune system. The sense organs that relate the brain to the environment, such as the eyes and ears, have parallels in a number of lymph organs. These are distinct regions that act as sensing devices and interact with stimuli: for example, patches in the intestine that constantly relate to what you eat.

Likewise, both systems have effectors. In the nervous system, these are typically the muscles that contract to produce behavior, although there are also other types. The equivalent in the immune system is the maturation of B-cells, an effect that is very important to health. In maturation, a B-cell suddenly changes state and becomes a factory producing about two thousand antibodies per hour instead of the usual dozen. These antibodies are released into the bloodstream independent of any cells; this effect is what we know as an immune response.

THE BODY'S SELF

We can now begin to look at a deeper analogy between the nervous system and the immune system. Just as the function of the nervous system takes on a cognitive identity, a sense of self, with its own memories, ideas, and tendencies, the body also has an identity or self with similar cognitive properties such as memory, learning, and expectations. This identity functions through the immune system.

The nervous system includes a number of simple mechanisms concerned with defending integrity. An animal avoids a painful stimulus; a driver turns the wheel to avoid a sudden collision. Biologists consider these emergency responses to be simple escape reflexes that happen at the lowest level of the nervous system, with very little sophistication. But the nervous system also has another side: all the emotion, imagination, desires, and memories that are part of ordinary life and are not concerned with urgent defense. There is a continuous inner life, an internal sense of identity, which is far more complex and interesting than simple escape reactions, and which involves most of the cortex.

In the immune system, we have exactly the same situation. The defensive aspects of the immune system respond to urgencies such as infection. For example, when bacteria enter the body, your immune system suddenly recognizes an unusual molecular entity. This recognition of an unfamiliar profile is a very simple cognitive operation. The B-cell clones that can bind to the bacteria start maturing and produce many, many antibodies. Each bacterium is completely surrounded by antibodies sticking to it, and is immediately washed away by fluids. This immune response is the basis of vaccines.[1]

The outer-directed defenses have dominated the study of immunology for 100 years, and awareness of the inner or autonomous aspect is very new, unlike in the neurosciences. Most immunology today is still concerned with immune responses, and it is based on the so-called Clonal Selection Theory, clearly formulated by MacFarland Burnet in the 1950s. I don't mean to imply that the immune response is not important. It is as necessary to life as are the neurological reflexes that propel one to run away from danger; but it would be silly to reduce our cognitive life to escape responses. Just as escaping danger and predators is only a small part of our cognitive life, we are often not confronted by serious infections. What happens to the immune system when there are no immune responses taking place? What is its equivalent of the inner cognitive life?

Let me use an analogy to illustrate the answer. What is the nature of the identity of a nation? France, for example, has an identity, and it is not sitting in the office of François Mitterand. Obviously, if too much of a foreign entity invades the system, it will have outer-directed defense reactions. The army mounts a military response. However, it would be silly to say that the military response is the whole of French identity. What is the identity of France when there is no war? Communication creates this identity, the tissue of social life, as people meet each other and talk. It is the life beat of the country. You walk in the cities and see people in cafes, writing books, raising children, cooking—but most of all, talking. Something analogous happens in the immune system as we construct our bodily identity. Cells and tissues have an identity as a body because of the network of B-cells and T-cells constantly moving around, binding and unbinding, to every single molecular profile in your body. They also bind and unbind constantly *among themselves*. A large percent of a B-cell's contacts are with other B-cells. Like a society, the cells build a tissue of mutual interaction, a functional network, as the work of several groups is showing. And it is through these mutual interactions, that lymphocytes are inhibited or expanded in clones, just as people get demoted or promoted, families expand or contract. This affirmation of a system's identity, which is not a defensive reaction but a positive construction, is a kind of self-assertion. This is what constitutes our "self" on the molecular and cellular level (including genetic determinants and "self" markers).

An experimental illustration that will make this more clear. Antonio Coutinho and his colleagues at Pasteur Institute in Paris raised mice in a bubble environment with no risk of infection, where they are exposed to no antigens (external molecules) other than air and very simple food. If you apply the classical view of the immune system as purely defensive, you would expect the mice to have no defense system. But if you see the immune system as having a cognitive inner core as well as outer defenses, you would expect these antigen-free mice to have a normal immune system. The results of the experiment are 100 percent clear: you can hardly differentiate between the immune systems of these antigen-free mice and those of mice raised normally. Obviously, outside of the chamber they will die, just as if you raised a child in an environment with no challenges, it would not know how to escape from danger. However, you can hardly distinguish its nervous system from that of a normal child. If a bubble mouse is gradually acquainted with antigens, it will survive—all it lacks is learning, essentially.

The classical view holds that antibodies are, just as the name suggests, directed against something else. It wouldn't make sense for them to bind to your own body. But in this alternative self-directed or network view of the immune system, dating back to the early seventies, from the work of Danish immunologist Niels Jerne, you would expect to find T-cells that can bind to every single molecular profile in the body. Just as for every aspect of French life—museums and libraries, cafes and pastries—there must be French people who deal with it. From the point of view of classical immunology, this is heresy. Paul Ehrlich, the founder of immunology, spoke of *horror autotoxicus,* the horror of responding to oneself. He saw the immune system as solely directed at invaders. The fact is, you do find antibodies to every single molecular profile in your body (cell membrane, muscle proteins, hormones, and so on). Instead of *horror autotoxicus,* there is a "know thyself" tendency between the immune system and the body. Through this distributed interdependence, a global balance is created, so that the molecules on my skin are in communication with the cells in my liver, because they are mutually affected via this circulating network of the immune system. From the perspective of network immunology, the immune system is nothing other than an enabler of the constant communication between every cell in your body, much as the neurons link distant places in the nervous system.

As I mentioned, the cells of the immune system die and are replaced roughly every two days, just as in a society people die after a number of years and children are constantly being born. Society in some complex way trains this pool of children to fill different roles. Similarly, the bone marrow is constantly producing what are known as infantile, or resting, B-cells. Some of these resting B-cells are recruited by the existing immune network and activated, or trained, to specific roles. This is how the system renews its components. Learning, or memory, happens because new cells are being "educated" into the system. The new cells are not identical to the old ones, but they fill the same role for the overall purpose of the emergent global picture.

The distinction between resting and active cells is important to the larger distinction between the outer-directed immune system, which is concerned with defenses, and the inner-directed immune system, which is concerned with molecular identity, or the assertion of the body's self. There is a close parallel here with the peripheral and central nervous systems; we can call them the peripheral immune system and the central immune system. The central immune system consists mostly of activated lymphocytes, which are larger and have more receptors on their surfaces. The peripheral immune system consists mainly of resting lymphocytes, which have fewer molecular profiles on the surface. So the two systems are distinguished not just metaphorically, but by criteria that are concrete and can be seen experimentally.

BRAIN-IMMUNE LINKS

Now that we've seen how this network of immune system interactions creates an identity in our body parallel to the cognitive identity of the nervous system's mind states, we can begin to ask how the immune system and the nervous system work together in the body. I want to give three examples that illustrate how these two selves work together.

The first experiments that convinced the scientific community that there was something to psychoneuroimmunology were done by psychologist Robert Ader. He used the notion of conditioning familiar to us from Pavlov's experiments with dogs. According to this theory, an actual stimulus (food) is replaced by a token stimulus (ringing a bell), and the salivation reaction still occurs. Ader assumed that if there was a neuroimmune connection, it would be possible to condition an immune reaction. He fed sugar water to rats, at the same time injecting them with psychophosphamine, a chemical that suppresses clones in the immune system. After repeating this for a while, the sugar water alone, without any drug, caused the suppression of clones. For this to be possible, there must be a way that the cognitive, perceptual act of tasting the sugar water affects the immune system. This is a clear example of psychoneuroimmunology, and it was very surprising to the scientific community.

A second example, also very recent, was the observation of a link between dyslexia and autoimmune diseases. Dyslexia appears as a learning problem in children who have trouble reading, which is a complex cognitive brain operation. They may see letters reversed, for example confusing *b* and *d*. Dyslexia is believed to be caused by problems in the early development of the brain, and we have known for years that dyslexic children show slight differences in brain physiology. Autoimmune diseases are caused when the immune system starts to treat a specific part of the body as if it were bacteria, and mounts an immune response to it. For example, in myasthenia gravis,[2] the immune system attacks the junctions between muscles and nerves, causing difficulty in movement as well as a lot of pain. There are many autoimmune diseases, and medical science has great difficulty dealing with them.

A few years back, it was shown that the great majority of children who have dyslexia also have autoimmune disorders. The two are clearly linked, and both can be traced to imbalances of certain hormones during development, particularly the gonadotrophic corticoid hormones. The same malfunction in the development of the nervous and immune systems can lead to related, but very distinct, effects. Again, this makes no sense from the standpoint of classical immunology.

The third example is the question of stress. Stress is obviously related to mind states and psychological attitude and also has a number of bodily effects. The question is, what are the pathways? The brain has been found to respond to stress very consistently and systematically by producing hormones such as glucocorticoids. These hormones are released into the bloodstream or directly into the lymphatic system. The hormones combine with the receptors on the surface of the lymphocytes, either suppressing them or activating them. As changes occur in the immune system, the lymphocytes also produce hormones and other messengers known as immunotransmitters. These molecules, in turn, directly affect specific neurons in the limbic system of the brain, so the link works in two directions.

Also very important is the finding that the autonomous nervous system, which is concerned with visceral control such as regulating the glands or the contraction of the muscles in the gut, can innervate the bone marrow. The autonomous nervous system grows directly into the bone marrow and can regulate the type and the number of T-cells produced there. The innervation of the bone marrow produces changes in the configuration of the immune system, which, in turn, causes the production of transmitters that effect changes in the brain. These are very clear and specific instances of neuroimmune interaction.

Scientists have also been able to trace other detailed examples of neuroimmune interactions that are very exciting. For instance, it has recently been found that some lymphocytes produce hormones called beta-endorphins. These are known as brain opiates, painkillers that are normally produced by the brain itself. So the same hormones that are transmitters inside the brain can be produced by lymphocytes, which in this case act as very distant neurons.

These are some of the pathways between the nervous system and the immune system that are becoming known. What is not known is how these effects can be more specific. For example, when we talk about immune suppression or activation, the effect is specific to certain clones. Likewise, the transmitters that suppress or stimulate neurons are known to affect specific sites of the brain. Obviously, the interactions between these two complex brains, the nervous system and the immune system, are specific, but how? This is an open question today. The fine tuning of the interactions between the two systems is not yet clear, but it is clear that these links do exist, and you can intervene in some ways to use them for medical purposes.

You might ask where the *psycho* part of psychoneuroimmunology comes in. Westerners, at least neuroscientists, make an automatic equation in their minds between emotional, perceptual, or cognitive states and neural activity. We tend to assume that a mental state involves measurable activity on the part of the brain, as, for example, when people feel stress, you can trace the pathways of the hormones that are released by the stressed brain. This psychoneuro correspondence is an important assumption in neuroscience.

Just as we have a neuropsycho identity, or parallel, there exists what I call the immunosoma, or immunobody identity. (There is an interesting language problem here. When I say *me,* I am using a designated label for what is mainly a psychological, cognitive complex. We don't even have a word in our language for the equivalent body, or *soma,* identity.) This immunobody has the same kind of wholeness or all-encompassing integrity that we have for our cognitive selves. For example, when I identify myself as me, Francisco, I am putting a label onto a complex. My body also labels itself in functioning. If I replace a little bit of my skin with another piece of skin, the tissue is rejected, even though I take pains to use exactly the same kinds of cells. The body recognizes it as not its own. If you could look inside the body, what appears to be simple tissue in fact sustains very active processes that are constantly going on, but are only revealed when challenged. We are not used to thinking of the body as a self that is as complex an entity as our cognitive selves, but the fact is that we do function that way, although we cannot consciously put a linguistic label on it.

Going back to the social analogy, I buy my bread every day from a baker in Paris whose family has been there for 200 years. He's part of the society, and he knows how to bake his bread. If suddenly one day I find a different person at the same bakery, who may be doing the same actions, selling the same bread, it still won't be the same. The baker belongs there because of the history of his long interactions, the fact that he's known people for a long time, and they have a common language. You can imitate this French baker, but if you don't have the right history and language and the capacity to interact, the neighbors will reject you too. What establishes my cells in their places and allows my liver cells to behave as liver cells, my thymus cells to behave as thymus cells, and so on, is the fact that they share this common language so they can operate in context with each other. Similarly, the baker knows the banker belongs to the community, even though the banker is doing something different.

We are so used to our body working that we don't appreciate the complexity of this emerging process that maintains its working. Much as in the human brain, where capacities such as memory or a sense of self are emergent properties of all the neurons, in the immune system there is an emergent capacity to maintain a body, and to have a history with it, to have a self. As an emergent property, it is something that arises but doesn't exist anywhere. From the point of view of psychoneuroimmunology, the body would also have an identity that is conceptually designated, but doesn't exist anywhere. My bodily identity is not localized in my genes or in my cells, but in the complex of the interactions.

DALAI LAMA: Is the presence of the immune system fundamentally the same even for extremely primitive organisms that have a neural system?

FRANCISCO VARELA: A very good question, Your Holiness, which I think clarifies the whole point. If you take a single-celled ameba, obviously there is no sense of an immune system. But when you have many cells coming together to form multicellular organisms, that is exactly where you see the beginnings of the immune system. Among primitive organisms, sponges have the simplest beginnings of an immune system.

DALAI LAMA: Do plants have some kind of immune system? Do they reject external materials?

FRANCISCO VARELA: They have other methods of defense, such as toxins. And single cells can ingest foreign molecules, so the immune system is not the only way to defend or to create an identity, but it is the way we vertebrates have done it.

DALAI LAMA: Do insects have an immune system?

FRANCISCO VARELA: Insects don't have an immune system. A fully developed immune system is unique to vertebrates.

DALAI LAMA: When the human body first forms, is it possible to say whether the immune system forms prior to the neural system or vice versa?

FRANCISCO VARELA: They form together. As I mentioned in the example of autoimmunity and dyslexia, when something goes slightly wrong in the embryo, both systems are affected. One becomes autoimmune, and tends to attack its own components; the other doesn't establish properly the cognitive property necessary for reading.

DALAI LAMA: Is it possible to say which of these two systems deteriorates first in the death process?

FRANCISCO VARELA: Brain death would take at most a few hours, from a biological standpoint. The connectivity of the immune system would break down as soon as circulation stopped. The lymphocytes would probably take, at most, a day to disappear. So they would both go pretty quickly.

DALAI LAMA: This may be the duration of their entire destruction, but do they begin simultaneously to deteriorate?

F R A N C I S C O V A R E L A :   In the process of death, the heartbeat would stop. That would cause anoxia to the brain; at the same time, the whole conversation that constitutes the immune system would stop, because without circulation the cells won't meet. Then the two kinds of cells, neurons and lymphocytes, would die within the next few hours. So the two systems are deteriorating pretty much in common. From the biological point of view, the identity of both systems would be dissolving. It would be body death, a soma death.

D A L A I L A M A :   When you have a bodily sensation such as pleasure, is there any involvement of the immune system?

F R A N C I S C O V A R E L A :   That's an open question. As we know, you can condition a form of immune suppression in response to a stimulus of sugar water, which is a perception of taste. There is no evidence against the idea that a pleasurable or unpleasant state could have specific immunomodulation effects, and in fact most of us believe that it does happen. It is also true that the experimental evidence is nonexistent, because transitory feeling is very hard to measure. We can only measure something that is very sustained, like stress.

D A L A I L A M A :   Is sensation entirely a matter of the nerves connecting and functioning properly? If you anaesthetize the body, or hypothetically remove all the nerves, would the bones and the flesh still have any capacity for feeling?

F R A N C I S C O V A R E L A :   As far as we know, if you cut or anaesthetize all the nerves coming to my hand, I will not have any more sensation of my hand. However, if that hand is accidentally burned, my soma mind or body mind knows it right away, and it reacts very intelligently. For example, it protects the wound by providing an inflammation reaction. It brings cells to repair and produce tissues. The immune system reacts by attempting to maintain harmony. So, while the mind of the nervous system is unaware of it, the other mind is responding intelligently.

DALAI LAMA: But the person would not be conscious of pain? This is a crucial point: when Buddhists speak of body awareness, the person is aware of the body.

FRANCISCO VARELA: I had understood body awareness in the Buddhist tradition as an awareness or a discriminatory faculty operating on the event, which is the body.

DALAI LAMA: Might there be a rough analogy if you damaged the leaf of the plant in some way? It doesn't feel anything or know anything, but it can take some defensive measures.

FRANCISCO VARELA: The analogy is rough, Your Holiness. The plant has only a simple capacity for regeneration. What our body can do is much more complex than that, and it is precisely that further complexity that gives it a higher state, that allows us to say that it's more like a mind than the simple immediate reflex of the plant tissues. The plant reacts in very limited ways that are almost always the same way, while our body has an enormous flexibility in maintaining itself.

DALAI LAMA: So the problem you were raising is, what is the identity of the body?

FRANCISCO VARELA: Yes. The fact is that the body has a wisdom to its own existence that entails regulation. If you take any hormone that circulates in your body, who controls the level of that hormone? To a large extent, the level is regulated by the immune system. For example, if my body is stressed as I'm exercising, the body by itself can recognize what it needs and decide what hormones to increase or decrease. All that wisdom happens without my linguistically conscious self knowing it, yet at the same time it is me in some important sense.

DALAI LAMA: You are saying that there are almost two parallel selves.

FRANCISCO VARELA: That's exactly my point. One is the self we're all used to and have a name for; the other one simply doesn't have any linguistic description, so we can see it only through its effects. But the wisdom of the body is an idea that belongs to many human traditions, and the interesting thing is that this neuroimmune connection might provide a more scientific angle on it.

DELUSION: PHYSIOLOGICAL AND MENTAL

DALAI LAMA: Why does the immune system sometimes attack its own family of cells and why are autoimmune diseases so deadly?

FRANCISCO VARELA: It's hard to say, but there are probably multiple causes. Some individuals are more prone to have autoimmune diseases. There seems to be a genetic component in many cases, but obviously that's not the whole story. Clearly, there are some weak links in the normal functioning of an individual, whether purely psychological or more on this "mind of the body" level.

The immune system allows us to have a bodily existence. If you interrupt the immune system you fall apart, even without infection in a protective bubble. Your body starts to disintegrate. This is actually what happens in the disease called lupus. Cells start to act without coordination, each in its own way. Coordinating a body with millions of different cells is an enormous job, just as much as coordinating a country with millions of people so that bakers continue to bake bread and bankers continue to do banking, and not the other way around. This coordinating role is the sense of the mind that we're talking about.

Traditional medicine, based on classical defense immunology, really doesn't know how to treat these autoimmune diseases, because they are examples of a slight disharmony in the sense of self. All of a sudden, one part that should be involved in the ongoing conversation somehow becomes a

foreigner. It's as if one group of people within a society becomes asocial, and their relationship with the society becomes aggressive. The appropriate treatment is nothing other
than to try to socialize them back, to provide more links with
society. Thus, some patients are cured with massive injections
of antibodies from a pool of donors.

Resocializing those parts of the body that have been ex-
cluded is exactly what has been attempted recently, with great
success, in mice with myasthenia gravis. By injecting B-cells
and antibodies that are known to provide further links between the existing immune system and the affected molecules,
in this case the muscle receptors, 90 percent of the mice were
cured. It is as if you provide new ways of opening a dialogue
with the asocial group so they can be harmonized back into
the body. So this whole process of harmonizing and regulating is cognitive, because it requires invention, memory, recognition, learning, and selective action. That's why I don't think
that it is exaggerating to speak about a second brain.

DALAI LAMA: Since the immune system can attack its
own family of cells, is it capable of healing the body?

FRANCISCO VARELA: It is impossible to think of
using the psychological mind, and therefore the brain, to heal
illness unless that mind is talking to another mind that is also
able to incorporate those messages in an intelligent way and
to regulate the body. Remission from cancer, for example,
must be an extremely complex phenomenon that requires an
intelligence in this immune system. We are never even conscious of it, but we see the effects constantly because we live
in our bodies. It inspires enormous awe and respect in me for
the complexity that exists in our organism and that we take
for granted.

DANIEL BROWN: Autoimmune disease, the body mis-
recognizing its own cells, is a kind of delusion from the
body's perspective. From the perspective of the mind, why
does delusion exist?

DALAI LAMA: Although Buddhism speaks of body
awareness, an awareness that resides within the body, delu-

sion can be present only as a mental cognition in which intelligence operates. So delusion cannot be present in sensory awareness, only in mental awareness. Delusion cannot be present at the sensory level, because that kind of cognitive intelligence doesn't work at the sensory level.

DANIEL BROWN: Why does delusion exist at the cognitive level?

DALAI LAMA: That's like asking: Why is there awareness? It just is.

SHARON SALZBERG: I wonder if there isn't a similarity to the autoimmune diseases, where the body doesn't recognize its own cells, its own integrity, and so begins to destroy itself. Perhaps an external version of that happens when, out of ignorance, we don't recognize others as ourselves. We start to destroy ourselves when we don't recognize our integrity, when we don't have a sense of all of life being like ourselves.

FRANCISCO VARELA: Interesting analogy.

DANIEL GOLEMAN: What we're getting to, it seems, is the idea that there is a Dharma of sorts to be learned from how cells behave—a biological basis for an ethical system.

NOTES

1. Vaccines are developed from fragments of viruses, killed viruses, or killed bacteria whose cell surfaces still retain the molecular markers unique to them. Once these neutralized infectious agents are introduced into the body via injection or, in some cases, by mouth, the immune system responds by producing antibodies to these molecular profiles. B-cell clones start to mature, and antibodies are made. The killed bacteria, virus, or virus fragment is treated by the immune system just like a live agent of infection. Thus, the body develops antibodies to a molecular profile it has not encountered through an actual infection. In a sense, vaccines create a mock

infection, a sort of fire drill that prepares the immune system before the actual threat occurs.

2. Myasthenia gravis is a chronic disorder of the muscles character-ized by weakness and a tendency to tire easily. Most commonly found in young adults, the disease is caused by a loss of muscle receptors for chemicals that induce muscle contraction. The mus-cles of the head and neck are most frequently involved.

4

The Brain and Emotions

CLIFF SARON AND
RICHARD J. DAVIDSON

A FLURRY OF findings in the last decade has given us a clearer picture than ever before of how the brain regulates emotions. It had long been assumed that the emotional centers were located deep within the brain in a series of structures that ring the underside of the cortex, called the limbic system (*limbic* is from the Latin for "ring"). More recent neurological data suggests that while emotional impulse originates in the limbic centers, how we *express* our emotions is regulated by structures that are newer in evolution, located in the prefrontal cortex just behind the forehead.

What's more, each side of the prefrontal cortex seems to handle a differing set of emotional responses, with more distressing emotions—those that might make us withdraw, say, in fear or disgust—regulated by the right side, and more positive feelings like happiness by the left. These neuroscience findings offer a backdrop for understanding the dynamics of our emotional lives. The emotions we feel, and how we handle them, are governed by this and other extensive and interconnected brain circuitry.

Cliff Saron reports on experiments done under the direction of his colleague, Richard Davidson, director of the Laboratory for Affective Neuroscience at the University of Wisconsin, that show in detail how the brain organizes aspects of our emotional reality. He begins by considering what "emotion" means, and explains how different theoretical models shape the methods used to study emotions and the brain. Then he reviews a series of key findings from their laboratory that offer new insights into how the brain regulates emotions like happiness and disgust, or more broadly, the tendencies to approach or withdraw—concepts parallel to Buddhist notions of attachment and aversion, the fundamental emotional poles that ground us in our worldly reality.

CLIFF SARON: What we mean by the word *emotion* is difficult to define in a strict sense. In psychology, the word is used to describe a person's responses at many different levels. One level is cognitive: the judgments and thoughts that arise in a particular feeling state. We can also describe emotion in terms of observed behavior: a gesture of anger or gentleness, a tone of voice. Facial expressions that spontaneously accompany moments of feeling are a particularly helpful way of specifying which emotion a person is feeling, and so constitute another way to define emotion.

On the physiological level, we can describe two components of emotional response: the body sensation that a person is aware of, such as a jittery feeling. Such sensations usually involve lower brain centers that control the autonomic nervous system and the release of hormones, with relatively long-lasting effects over a period of minutes or hours. A second physiological response is in the cerebral cortex. That's the level of emotional response our work focuses on.

We also look at approach and withdrawal as fundamental ways of describing the behavior of an organism and categorizing different emotions. For example, happiness may move you toward someone you're very glad to see. Fear and disgust are typical examples of withdrawal behavior. This approach and withdrawal behavior can be linked to activity on each side of the brain. Over the last ten years, we have produced a series of results in our laboratory suggesting that the front regions of the left side of the brain are more associated with approach behavior, and those of the right side are more associated with withdrawal behavior.

You could ask why we would ever want to relate approach and withdraw behavior to the two sides of the brain. It's not an obvious relationship. But information from neurology over the last hundred years indicates that damage to each side of the brain has different emotional consequences.

In the mid-nineteenth century, the neurologist John Hughlings Jackson noted that people who suffered from epileptic seizures, which begin with too much activity in the right frontal regions of the brain, consistently expressed fear—a withdrawal emotion—at the onset of their seizures. Patients with damage resulting in too little activity on the right side of the brain, however, experienced manic or inappropriately positive emotions. These observations gave rise to a theory about how the two sides of the brain may have different emotional specializations or characters. Overactivation of the right side of the brain seems to enhance withdrawal behavior; and when the right side is depressed or damaged, approach behavior is enhanced because the left side has the majority of control, without the balance of the right side.

Two other, very different ways of thinking about emotion are a point of controversy in psychology. One view is that there are a few discrete basic emotions: happiness, sadness, anger, disgust, surprise, and fear. A little over twenty years ago, Paul Ekman at the University of California at San Francisco documented the universality of facial expressions in different cultures. His work was inspired by Darwin's book *The Expression of Emotion in Man and Animals*. Ekman studied facial expressions of Westerners and of a preliterate tribe in New Guinea who had virtually no contact with Western culture. By asking people to identify pictures of facial expressions and to make their own facial expression for emotions they defined themselves, he found that the expression of certain basic emotions was similar in both cultures.

This model of discrete emotions is challenged by the dimensional view: that specific emotional states represent locations along a continuum, which might range from approach to withdrawal, or from pleasantness to unpleasantness. Both the discrete and dimensional views are current in scientific psychology, and our work draws on elements of both, since neither seems complete in itself.

The methods we use to measure emotion in a particular experiment implicitly draw on these models. If we ask people to evaluate how pleasant or unpleasant they feel, we're using the dimensional approach. If we analyze facial expressions specific to happiness or disgust, then we're applying a discrete view. We can't simultaneously analyze all the different aspects that are included in our definition of emotion, any more than we can simultaneously locate all the immune cells in the body.

Our experiments simplify this complexity quite a bit. We've taken three different approaches to studying the relationship between brain activity and emotion. The first, very basic approach is to bring a person into the laboratory and, hopefully, elicit specific emotional reactions while we measure his or her brain activity. A second approach is to evaluate a large number of people and identify those who differ in emotional functions such as temperament or depression, and examine whether they also differ in terms of their brain activity. The third approach is the converse of this. We take people who differ consistently in their brain activity and examine whether they differ in terms of their emotional functioning. Our experiments include each type of approach.

CAPTURING EMOTIONS IN THE LABORATORY

In one experiment, we brought people into our laboratory and showed them films designed to elicit specific emotions. We showed happy films—a puppy playing with a flower, a gorilla taking a bath at the zoo—and we showed films that arouse negative emotions—medical training films of a third-degree-burn victim and of surgical amputation of a leg. We used these particular films because the facial expressions they elicit had already been studied by Paul Ekman, who collaborated with us on this project. As the subjects were watching the films, we videotaped their facial expressions and simultaneously recorded their brain activity. Using a system for coding emotion from facial expressions, we can tell if people are feeling, for example, disgust or happiness. Interpretation of these expressions is not based on our opinions of what disgust or happiness look like, but on years of research by Paul Ekman defining the basic facial characteristics that people rate as best representing a specific emotion.

When you're using the face as an indicator of emotion, you need to be aware of three possibilities. You can have an expression with no feeling, a feeling with no expression, or an expression that is not pure. For example, there can be different forms of a smile depending on the social circumstance. It might also be hard for certain people to produce certain expressions. Some people inhibit the expression of anger, for example, even when they're alone. You have to be sure that the stimulus can actually elicit the expressions you want to examine. So we use the films to elicit emotion and a videotape of the viewers' facial expressions to measure it.

The third ingredient, measuring the brain, is a little more complicated. We use a special cap to record an electroencephalograph (EEG), measuring very small amounts of electrical activity at different regions on the surface of the head. This actually represents only a small portion of brain activity; it's very different from listening to a heartbeat through a stethoscope.

The electrical signal is the combined activity of many millions of nerve cells, and their "noise" is a property we can take advantage of. When a given region of the cortex is not actively engaged in processing information, it produces oscillations at a frequency of about ten cycles per second. From moment to moment, the electrical activity changes, and this characteristic oscillation appears at different locations on the surface of the brain, depending on the type of mental activity that the person is engaged in at that moment. It's a very dynamic and rapidly changing phenomenon.

There is a distinction between the gross electrical activity that we measure in voltages and its significance for the operation of the brain. More voltage does not necessarily mean more activity; you have to look at the whole pattern. For example, people used to think that when light enters the eye it would make the photo-pigment cells more active. When finally it was possible to measure their electrical activity, it turned out that light makes these cells *less* active. In this case, a decrease in voltage—less electrical activity—signifies there is something to be seen—more involvement.

At any rate, when nerve cells are at rest, they make a characteristic pattern of oscillations. When nerve cells receive input and are busy communicating information from one location to another, the oscillations stop. We measured these electrical oscillations during facial expressions of happiness and disgust. We had asked people to rate their experience after seeing the films, so the results were normalized to reflect equal intensities of happiness and disgust. The clearest difference between the two facial expressions was that the right frontal region was more involved during disgust.

Each person we measured had increased right hemisphere involvement during disgust as compared to happiness, even though the increase might have been slight. But people differed widely in terms of their brain activity even normally, when they were just sitting and resting. For those at one end of the range, the left side was always more activated than the right, even during disgust. At the other end of the range, the right side was always more activated than the left, even during happiness. So we were dealing with subtle changes and a broad range of individual differences.

Emotions in Children: Innate Patterns

We wanted to find out if these differences in right and left brain activity are learned or are present from birth. So we did a similar experiment with newborns between one and three days old. We didn't show them the same movies, but we did look at brain activity that accompanied different facial expressions. We gave the babies a taste of sweet sugar water, and a taste of sour lime juice. It's impossible to know what they were actually feeling, but we described the facial expression in response to the sweetness as interest, while the sour taste seemed to elicit disgust.

Using a little electrode cap, we measured electrical activity of the front and rear regions of the brain. The results for newborn babies were very similar to those of adults in the previous experiment. The right frontal region became more involved during the disgust expression, and there was a slight change in the left rear during interest. These results demonstrated this phenomenon is part of our biological makeup, not socially acquired.

In the nineteenth century, a French anatomist named Duchenne of Bologne analyzed the muscles of the face and observed that a genuine expression of happiness has two components. During a genuinely felt smile, a muscle around the eyes tightens, causing little crows' feet. A second muscle involved in a smile is the cheek muscle—called the dimpler—that pulls the lips out into a smile. By applying an electric current to this muscle, Duchenne found he could make the muscle contract to produce a nongenuine smile.

Our research used this understanding in another experiment, this time with ten-month-old babies, in collaboration with Nathan Fox, a developmental psychologist. We videotaped each child, seated on a chair, while his or her mother approached, and the child smiled. But when a stranger approached, the children more often showed the unfelt smile, without the involvement of the eyes.

In work with adults, we compared activity in the front and rear regions on both sides of the brain during felt and unfelt smiles. During unfelt smiles there was an increase in right hemisphere involvement in the front regions, and during felt smiles there was more left hemisphere involvement. The difference was much bigger in the front part of the brain than it was in the rear region. Remember that the felt smiles were elicited by the mother's approach, so again the notion of approach and withdrawal is applied to brain states. And, when the babies displayed the felt smiles, they also showed a dramatic increase in left-sided frontal activity compared to the activity registered by unfelt smiles.

THE DEPRESSIVE TENDENCY

Our second approach to the study of emotion separated people on the basis of their emotional functioning and then looked at their differences in brain activity. In this next experiment we considered individuals who were depressed, because people with damage to the left side of the brain are especially vulnerable to depression. If the left side is damaged, it no longer counterbalances the activity of the right side, so there is a greater possibility of experiencing negative emotional states more often.

We compared depressed people with a nondepressed control group, measuring their brain activity while they just sat quietly with their eyes open for three minutes and again with their eyes closed. We were looking for differences, or asymmetry, in resting activity between the right and left frontal regions.

For the depressed group, the right hemisphere was more active than the left hemisphere, but for the control group the left hemisphere was more active than the right. So the basic finding was that in a group of people who are deficient in their ability to feel approach emotions like happiness, there is less activation of the left frontal region compared to the right. Another way to think of this is that the withdrawal system is more activated than the approach system.

These brain differences are not always related to a person's emotional states at the moment. In another experiment, the people we looked at had a history of depression but were not currently depressed. Their frontal brain asymmetry was very similar to that of currently depressed people. These findings suggest that the differences in resting asymmetry between the left and right sides of the brain represent a tendency of emotional response rather than the emotional response itself. Indeed, other experiments show that we can *predict* how happy or sad a person will feel in response to a film, just on the basis of the resting asymmetry of the two hemispheres.

THE INHIBITED TEMPERAMENT

As a dimension of temperament, some children are very uninhibited and actively approach their environment. Others are more inhibited or wary; they stay closer to their mothers and play less with other children. In another experiment, we were interested in seeing whether these temperamental differences in children would show up as differences in brain activity.

We studied 368 children who were two-and-a-half years old. We brought each child to the laboratory for a play session in a room full of toys, along with his or her mother and another mother and child. We timed how long it took the child to leave the mother's side and approach the toys, and also tracked when the child first spoke and how much the child talked. We also introduced a talking toy robot into the room, and later a stranger, and recorded whether the children approached or withdrew from them.

We identified thirty of the most uninhibited, outgoing children, who were by their mothers' side less than 1 percent of the time; and the thirty most wary, fearful children, who stayed by their mothers at least 80 percent of the time. We also selected a group of thirty from the middle of the range. To see whether these groups differed in their brains' electrical activity, we brought them into the lab and measured their EEG while they were sitting as quietly as possible. To get them to sit still, we told them they were going to be racing car drivers, and put them in a toy car with the EEG cap as a racing helmet.

We found that the two groups differed in their resting brain activity. The uninhibited children, who were eager to approach the toys, showed a pattern of greater left hemisphere involvement. The inhibited children, who were more withdrawn, showed greater right hemisphere involvement. The results from the middle group were midway between the other two.

The main difference between these groups was the level of activity in the left hemisphere, while the activity level on the right side was not meaningfully different. The inhibited children showed decreased activity on the left frontal region, presumably reflecting an underactive approach system. In the very outgoing, uninhibited group, the left frontal region showed far more activation. So the involvement is apparently a function of temperament.

BRAIN AND TEMPERAMENT

Finally, we classified people on the basis of their brain activity and then examined whether they differed emotionally. We wanted to know if people who have more activation of the left frontal regions are generally happier, and whether people with more right frontal activity experience more negative emotion. We tested about a hundred people for several minutes over two sessions, because individuals can vary in response at different times.

We selected two groups who had consistently shown the most extreme activation of the left or right side on both occasions. We then asked them to fill out a questionnaire describing how they generally felt in terms of positive emotions—happy, sad, proud, confident, outgoing, helpful—or various negative emotions.

The people who had greater activation of the left anterior region showed more positive emotions about their lives, in general, or in response to challenges, whereas those with more active right hemispheres showed more negative emotional responses. So people appear to differ in emotional quality even when selected only on the basis of resting brain activity. We can't really say what comes first, but if there is persistent activity on the right side of the brain, there's a probability that a person may feel generally worse during their daily life activities than someone whose left side is more activated.

If that's true, there might be health consequences to persistent negative emotions accompanied by persistent involvement of the right hemisphere. To see whether people selected only on the basis of their EEG differed in their immune response, we tested their blood for a certain component of the immune system.

The cytotoxicity of killer cells—their effectiveness in destroying foreign elements—was greater for the group with more left hemisphere activity. We do not know that this group is healthier, but the data suggest they would be. We are in the process of determining whether or not such people in fact have a better health history, though it is unlikely any difference in health would emerge until later in life.

EMOTIONAL REACTIVITY: A FINAL NOTE

There is evidence suggesting that other brain structures are very important in controlling emotional experience, the amygdala being one. These structures are not in the cerebral cortex but at a lower level in the brain's organization. A path of communication has been worked out by Joseph LeDoux, a neuroscientist at New York University, showing that sensory information can take two separate paths: one up to the cortex and another through the thalamus to the amygdala. The connection to the amygdala is very quick—a direct connection—but not very precise, because most of the sensory information goes via the other path, up to the neocortex, where it is analyzed through several circuits while a response is formulated.

But the amygdala, meanwhile, quickly assesses the sensory data to see if it has emotional meaning and can trigger a response while the neocortex is still sorting things out. Emotions may be very difficult to control because the amygdala turns on other parts of the brain before the thinking brain, the neocortex, does.

Because the amygdala has diverse connections to parts of the brain that control the autonomic nervous system, as well as connections to the cortex, which is responsible for conscious experience, there is a hypothesis that the amygdala serves as a place of convergence, giving it a central role in emotional life, so it can mobilize the body to respond with a strong emotion, particularly fear, before the thinking brain quite knows what's happening.

Scientists have discovered that there is an anatomical connection between the frontal cortex and the amygdala. From recent experiments, it appears that one important function of this connection is for the frontal cortex to regulate or turn off the amygdala. For example, we might be frightened by something moving in the night that we cannot quite see clearly. However, once we see that it is something innocuous, we can inhibit the fear that was just previously generated. The prefrontal cortex appears to play an important role in this type of regulation. Those individuals with more left-sided frontal activation may be better at turning off their amygdalas once they get activated so that negative emotions do not linger.

DALAI LAMA: In other words, there is preconscious activation in the brain that triggers emotions, and only afterward are you actually aware of what's going on?

CLIFF SARON: Yes, that is what I am suggesting. There is actually some very recent data that humans with damage to the right amygdala were unable to experience appropriate negative emotions. But their left amygdala was fine, and they had normal positive emotions.

DALAI LAMA: Well, that's good!

CLIFF SARON: But I don't think we should go scooping out everybody's right amygdala!

DALAI LAMA: When you say that certain emotions, such as happiness, are good for the physical health, and others, such as disgust, are bad for the health, does this directly pertain to the amount of brain activity in different parts of the brain?

CLIFF SARON: Differences in brain activity can be associated with differences in the immune system, but we do not know whether these differences affect health. That is an important distinction.

DALAI LAMA: Is it true to say that the body's harmony or equilibrium is not disturbed by wholesome emotions such as happiness, but that in the case of unwholesome emotions such as hatred, the intensified activity disturbs the equilibrium? Could we say that more activity in certain parts of the brain would be detrimental because it disturbs the equilibrium?

CLIFF SARON: It is partly true. It's important to remember that equilibrium is actually very dynamic. There's no perfect state. We could have an interesting discussion about perfection and equilibrium, but biological systems are very, very dynamic. There may be an equally great disturbance during positive emotions: the term *disturbance* has an inappropriately negative connotation. It is true, however, that the right side of the brain influences other structures that secrete hormones associated with increased breakdown of parts of the body. If the right side of the brain is habitually overactive, there can be a relationship between habitual negative emotional states and an increased secretion of unwholesome chemicals.

EMOTIONS AND CULTURAL CATEGORIES

CLIFF SARON: Earlier, we were talking about universal emotions that have facial expressions associated with them. I was wondering whether in Buddhist psychology there is a group of feeling states, or whatever term you would use as equivalent to emotions, that are limited in number but for which different combinations are sufficient to account for much of our experience?

DALAI LAMA: You're asking whether there are any fundamental emotions. When you introduce an alien term, and therefore an alien concept, into the Buddhist framework, then it is very hard to respond. There is no word in Tibetan that can be translated as "emotion" in English. However, if you speak of one category of emotion, like negative emotions—*kleshas*, or afflictions—then definitely there are six primary ones, but even here it is tricky to use the English word *emotion*. The six prominent ones are ignorance, attachment, anger, pride, wrong views, and skepticism or afflictive doubt.

The terminology becomes doubtful when you call ignorance an emotion; and within ignorance there are different categories. There is a sort of ignorance that is simply a dullness or lack of clarity, and to call that an emotion would be very, very tenuous. On the other hand, there are more dynamic forms of ignorance that entail a false mode of apprehending reality. Possibly you could call them emotions.

CLIFF SARON: Your Holiness, I wonder if there's any way to relate the type of ignorance that grasps at phenomena as truly relating to the concept of emotions and their role in attachment?

DALAI LAMA: The term *emotion* has gotten so nebulous by now that it's difficult to talk about. We've already decided that the Buddha has emotions. If you look at negative emotions—attachment, hostility, and such things—then there's definitely a relationship between the grasping onto phenomena as truly existent and these emotions. That is to say, such emotions as attachment or hatred arise on the basis of grasping the given object as being truly existent. If you're attached to something, that attachment will arise on the basis of grasping it as truly existent. If you hate a certain object, that hate will arise on the basis of grasping that object as being truly or inherently existent.

Here's an example: Imagine that you're feeling terribly angry at a person named John. As you're focusing your anger upon John, what are you angry at? You're just angry at John himself. This inherently existing John is the object of your anger. If someone challenges you and says, "Where is John? Is John his body, or is John his mind?" don't you have a sense that somehow you've lost your target a little bit? You're taken aback. There's a corollary explanation for attachment.

LEE YEARLEY: Why can't I just say that I'm angry at John's arrogance, or his selfishness? It's not related to John's body or John's compassion; it's just a quality of his that I hate.

DALAI LAMA: That's fine! [*laughter*] It's fine to have that attitude toward John's faults, because that's authentic, as long as simultaneously you're wishing that John might meet with well-being and be free of suffering.

SHARON SALZBERG: Are all the emotions approach or avoidance?

CLIFF SARON: Not every emotion is an example of approach or withdrawal, but in scientific research it has been a helpful way to think about emotions in general.

DALAI LAMA: So would you say that attachment or craving on the one hand, and hostility or aversion on the other, are primary emotions? What about doubt? Or equanimity? Would you say that equanimity is a point of no emotion or a neutral emotion? How do you distinguish between emotions and other cognitive activity? What are the parameters?

CLIFF SARON: Our common-sense vocabulary is a central problem in talking about emotions. In terms of Western scientific psychology, doubt is not considered a basic emotion, like anger, happiness, or sadness. However, it is certainly a feeling state that we can identify. When you say "doubt," I know what you mean.

DALAI LAMA: Take, for instance, a person who first experiences a quandary of doubt. It could be a scientist. [*laughter*] But then, by applying reason and drawing on experimental evidence, this person cuts through the doubt and comes to a very clear sense of conviction. Is that strong feeling of certainty and full conviction an emotion or not?

CLIFF SARON: Certainty, confidence, and pride would be considered emotions.

DALAI LAMA: Is the certainty itself an emotion, or does an emotion arise simultaneously with the certainty?

CLIFF SARON: It's possible you could feel neutral about the results of experiments that are conclusively true. However, scientists, as people committed to research, have very strong cravings for answers. You can be very attached to your hypothesis, and feel an emotional rush when it is proven true.

DALAI LAMA: I'm not referring simply to some kind of attachment or craving, but actually the inferential insight that arises in one's mind, sometimes very emphatically, on the basis of the preceding reasoning. Suppose your hypothesis is proven wrong. This may lead to a sense of disappointment, but the results of your experiments are unequivocal and you feel completely certain. Is that also an emotional state?

CLIFF SARON: The disappointment is the emotional state. The insight that you were wrong is not an emotional state.

DALAI LAMA: So you would say that the cognitive ascertainment itself is not an emotion, but the emotion, whether it is exaltation or depression, arises simultaneously with the ascertainment?

CLIFF SARON: Yes. The emotion is the feeling that arises in response to whatever triggers it. In this case we're talking about a scientist's experience, but it could also be winning or losing the lottery. The situation is also unequivocal, and you could feel the same kind of exaltation or disappointment.

DALAI LAMA: It looks rather like emotion is reduced to either pleasure or displeasure. Is it more than that? What is an emotion?

DANIEL BROWN: An emotion has at least three necessary components: the felt bodily experience, the cognition or thought, and an expressive reaction. If you have just the bodily sense without the thought, for example, then it's not an emotion because the thought helps distinguish the kind of emotion. If you have just a thought without a bodily sense, that's not an emotion either.

DALAI LAMA: Aren't there cases of people whose bodies have lost sensation? Are those people bereft of emotions? Wouldn't somebody who is completely paralyzed and without bodily feeling still experience fear?

FRANCISCO VARELA: It's clear that people who have been paralyzed still feel emotion. Although we normally associate emotions with the bodily feelings, the cognitive part alone could suffice for the experience of emotion even though the neurotransmitters may not be able to bring the visceral effects into awareness. So, although there are normally three components, you could still have a relatively valid emotion if one of the three were weakened.

DANIEL BROWN: Yes, one dimension could carry more weight than others.

CLIFF SARON: Paul Ekman is studying several people with Bell's palsy, a paralysis that prevents facial expression. Others may have no idea what such people are feeling when they interact, but they do feel very intensely. It would be entirely possible to show experimentally that the brain changes corresponding to emotions in a normal person are similar to those in a person unable to express the feeling. However, emotion is a very complex concept, because it involves not just the three components but also the relationships between them and their order in time. Do I identify an emotion, such as fear, because I recognize certain bodily changes? There's a whole school of emotion theory that thinks in terms of preconscious reactions setting off body reactions that then inform conscious awareness.

SHARON SALZBERG: In listening to the presentation the thought came to me that, in the Buddhist system, both the approach and withdrawal emotions Cliff described can be wholesome or unwholesome. We can have a wholesome approach emotion toward an object, such as a face, that draws us close, or we can have an unwholesome approach emotion such as greed. Likewise, we can have an unwholesome avoidance such as laziness, or a very wholesome withdrawal as when conscience restrains us from an action.

DALAI LAMA: There can also be a wholesome mental state that is concomitant with a feeling of equanimity. Where would that fit into this system? [pause] Why doesn't anybody respond from neuroscience?

DANIEL GOLEMAN: Well, one can approach or avoid with equanimity. I think that this system can't handle equanimity; it doesn't fit.

FRANCISCO VARELA: I would like to reiterate the point that avoidance and approach are only one dimension in the study of emotion from a neurophysiological point of view. This is not at all exhaustive, but it's relatively easy. It's like studying people who are awake or asleep; that doesn't mean those are the only two mental states, but they offer a dramatic contrast. So there is no attempt here to make everything fit. There are many things that won't fit. Part of the problem, also, is that there is no agreed-upon classification of emotions or definition of what an emotion is. To a large extent in the West an emotion happens to be what you can measure. A psychological method will measure and classify emotions differently from a linguistic approach. If you measure brain activity, you notice avoidance reactions, but if you measure hormonal release of adrenaline, you find another set of categories.

DANIEL BROWN: The trouble is, it's hard to measure the subjective feeling state. It's easier to measure the expressive facial display and its relation to brain activity, so science is more involved in this.

FRANCISCO VARELA: Would it be possible, Your Holiness, to have a cognition without an emotion? Or without a mental affliction, a disturbing emotion?

DALAI LAMA: It's certainly possible to have a cognition without a mental affliction. However, for any kind of cognition there will be some feeling, whether it is pleasurable, unpleasant, or one of indifference.

FRANCISCO VARELA: Is there any emotionlike tone, other than feeling?

DALAI LAMA: Feeling is one of five omnipresent mental factors, and the one that is the closest to being translatable as "emotion. "

FRANCISCO VARELA: I'm asking the question because in the West, there is a tendency to imagine that one could have cognition without any emotional tonality. The most typical example is the robots that people have imagined in science fiction, which are very intelligent and have many cognitive qualities. They can infer, deduct, remember, and generalize, yet they are completely without feelings or emotions. I think they represent an expression of the view that emotion does not necessarily enter into cognition, that these two things can be disassociated.

DALAI LAMA: I would speculate that if they did in fact have cognition, they probably would have feeling as well.

DANIEL BROWN: Feeling, but not emotion?

ALAN WALLACE: Tibetan doesn't have a word for emotion.

The Importance of Equanimity in Tibetan Buddhism

DALAI LAMA: Is there a school of thought that says equanimity is not an emotion and happiness and sadness are?

CLIFF SARON: Equanimity is not a word that Western psychologists have spent a lot of time discussing.

DANIEL GOLEMAN: Or experiencing. [*laughter*]

ROBERT THURMAN: Could bliss consciousness be considered an emotion?

DALAI LAMA: That would be an emotion, a big one! [*laughter*]

FRANCISCO VARELA: Could I ask for a clarification, Your Holiness? Would the tranquility or equilibrium of the mind be considered like a reference state? Is there something like an ideal state of mind? Or is it not the case that mind could be many multiple states which could be perhaps not restful, could be very active, but—

ALAN WALLACE: The opposite of peaceful is not active.

FRANCISCO VARELA: That's what I wanted to understand. It sounds from the initial translation as if there was this reference point of serenity, tranquility, equilibrium, but it's difficult to see how that could also be an active life.

DALAI LAMA: I feel that possibly the very nature of the mind is equanimity. That is, the feeling that normally accompanies a natural state of mind is that of equanimity. Normally when we rest, we try to just rest without having any conscious thoughts, but at that time we are not trying to stop any thoughts. So, what we're trying to do is to remain in a natural state of mind with the feeling of equanimity. It's when you have mental afflictions that the equilibrium is disturbed.

FRANCISCO VARELA: But in the moment when you're not sitting, when you are buying bread or talking to somebody on your job, can you still have that equanimity? It seems like there is no way to be in equanimity unless one is sitting down.

ALAN WALLACE: The etymology of the Tibetan word translated as mental affliction means "that which afflicts the mind." You might be mentally very active without the mind being afflicted. It's active, and yet has an equilibrium in the senseof not being afflicted.

FRANCISCO VARELA: So it is not a unique state that requires inactivity. That's what I was trying to get at, because serenity normally is associated with inactivity.

DALAI LAMA: As you cultivate compassion and the desire to be free, they do in fact disturb the mind. But you can get around that as a problem by looking at the long-term effects. Bear in mind that there are subtle differences among various schools of thought as to which states of mind are afflictive, based on the differences in theories of emptiness, which is the Buddhist understanding of the nature of reality. A certain state of mind may be seen from the Prasangika point of view as an afflictive mental state, but for another school of thought it may be perfectly sound. For example, as we look at a flower and apprehend it as existing in its own right, the Prasangika school would say that this mode of apprehending it is a mental affliction. But for every other philosophical school within Buddhism apart from Prasangika, that mode of apprehension is considered perfectly authentic, because they say the flower does exist in its own right. Because of the difference of opinion regarding the nature of subtle ignorance, then implicitly there's also a difference of opinion about the nature of subtle attachment and subtle anger.

5

Stress, Trauma, and the Body

DANIEL BROWN

"STRESS" IS SO common a part of our late twenti-
eth-century vocabulary that its meaning is sometimes obscured. Technically speaking, a stress reaction is a mental
and physical response to an adverse situation that mobilizes the body's emergency resources, the "fight or flight"
mechanism, which floods the body with hormones that
arouse it to meet the challenge. Unfortunately, modern life
continually triggers this response when we can neither fight
nor flee, which can lead to chronic heightening of blood
pressure and muscle tension, irritability, anxiety, and depression—and a lowering of immune effectiveness.

Daniel Brown explores how stress leads to particular illnesses. His perspective is behavioral medicine, a relatively
new branch of medicine that applies behavioral methods,
including biofeedback, meditation, and hypnosis, to the
treatment of chronic illnesses and the promotion of ways
to prevent illness. Brown discusses internal and external
triggers of illness; he explains how stress affects the functioning of the nervous system and describes the cumulative
effect on the body of chronic stress.

There are various ways of coping with distress. Some ways of coping with stress—substance abuse, for example—lead to greater problems; others, like biofeedback and meditation, promote resiliency and improved health. The pressures and disturbing events of our lives need not dictate how the body and mind respond.

Perhaps the most severe effect of intense stress is found in posttraumatic stress disorder (PTSD). This psychological disorder typically develops in people who have experienced extreme forms of trauma, such as torture, sexual abuse, combat, or a life-threatening event like an auto accident or a hurricane. Symptoms include recurrent flashbacks of the traumatic event, nightmares, eating disorders, anxiety, fatigue, and social withdrawal. People with PTSD have an overactive stress response, which triggers intense arousal of the autonomic nervous system in response to benign, ordinary situations. The Dalai Lama points out that as a result of their meditative training, some Tibetan refugees and monks who have been incarcerated by the Chinese have coped amazingly well, seemingly without PTSD, even under the direst mistreatment.

DANIEL BROWN: Behavioral medicine brings together the wisdom of psychology and medical science in understanding how to assess and diagnose illness, how to treat it, and particularly how to prevent it, as well as rehabilitation. It has been applied more or less successfully in a variety of areas, particularly the treatment of psychophysiological disorders, such as headache, pain, hypertension, and asthma. The second area is the use of these methods in approaching health-risk behavior, such as smoking, poor sleeping habits, or poor eating habits—behavior in which a person's ordinary habits affect his or her health in a negative way.

The third area of behavioral medicine is the understanding of how people adjust to chronic illness, such as diabetes or kidney disease. For example, many diabetics don't adhere to their prescribed medical treatment. They eat very poorly and don't watch their blood sugar levels, or neglect the schedule for taking their insulin, even though they know the treatment will work. So scientists began to study this whole issue of compliance as part of a patient's adjustment to chronic illness.

The fourth area is more controversial: the use of these methods in the prevention and treatment of immune-related illnesses, such as cancer, AIDS, and autoimmune disease. That is a less-developed field. The fifth area of treatment is traditionally known as psychosomatic medicine: the connection between the mind and the body, and the use of behavioral methods in the treatment of such things as anxiety-induced medical symptoms like asthma attacks.

Lastly, behavioral medicine has been applied to what is now called wellness enhancement. This is not so much treating illness, but preventing it in the first place by teaching methods for achieving an optimal state of health.

ILLNESS: CAUSES AND MAINTENANCE

In behavioral medicine, it's important to start with some understanding of how we view illness and the development of illness. In our clinic, we look at illness on two levels: first in terms of causation and then in terms of different factors that maintain the illness. The causes of illness may be biological, or stress related, or both. Biological factors include genetic predisposition, as for example in autoimmune disease and some forms of cancer. Other causative factors are things that happen in a person's early life. The pattern of early nutrition, for example, may affect weight later in life. Sometimes early infections can cause tissue damage; pneumonia in the first year of a baby's life may make the lung tissue more sensitive later to the development of asthma. Sometimes people acquire a sensitivity to certain drugs. In some people with asthma, the asthma is caused by an acquired sensitivity. Sometimes, people have an injury that has lasting results, and this is important in the development of illness later in life. These are all examples of biological causes that predispose a person to developing illness.

Second, we look at the factors that maintain illness, because the research has increasingly made clear that the factors that maintain an illness over a period of time may be different from the factors that originally caused it. Just as it is possible to condition or train a response from the immune system, the same kind of thing happens with asthma: people can have asthma attacks as a learned response. Anticipatory anxiety is another factor that can maintain illness. For example, some asthmatics worry about an asthma attack coming on. The worry causes changes in the autonomic nervous system, which then cause changes in the lung tissue, producing an asthma attack. Overuse of certain treatments is another factor, particularly sprays that offer short-term relief from an attack, but which leave lung tissue even more exposed to the substances that inflame them to trigger the asthmatic attack. The very treatment maintains the illness rather than making it go away.

These factors that maintain the illness are separate from the causes; the illness takes on a life of its own and becomes complex. It's important to treat both the causes and the conditions that maintain the illness, so we look at the development of illness as complex.

STRESS AND THE AUTONOMIC NERVOUS SYSTEM

Behavioral scientists have focused on the relation of stress to illness development and an understanding of the autonomic nervous system. The autonomic nervous system controls functions like muscle tension and heart rate. It also controls the vasomotor response by controlling the muscles around the tubing of the blood vessels so they expand or contract to redirect the blood throughout the body at various times. When you're digesting your food after breakfast, the blood vessels in the stomach area expand so that more blood goes to that area. When you're doing effort-ridden thinking, like reading, the blood vessels in the head expand. When you're very relaxed, the capillaries in the skin expand and distribute the blood throughout the skin.

The autonomic nervous system is an emergency defense system. One aspect of the defense reaction is the classic fight-or-flight response. When the organism is threatened, there is usually an arousal, along with increased muscle tension, to prepare one either to run away or to strike out to defend oneself. Heart rate increases and the blood vessels in the skin contract. The blood is redirected to the muscles and to the brain to make the organism more alert, to prepare for action. We observe this classic fight-or-flight reaction in animals and in humans in times of threat, but the autonomic arousal is more elaborate in humans. We also see less intense forms of it in ordinary activities during the day. For example, the same pattern of increased heart rate, decreased size of the blood vessels in the skin, and increase in muscle activation occurs when we concentrate mentally, preparing to act. Any kind of preparation or readiness for action is accompanied by this autonomic activation with changes in the muscle tension level and the blood flow. Both the fight-or-flight reaction and its lesser version, the activation for alertness and readiness to perform as we move around and think and engage the world, are aspects of the autonomic nervous system. These reactions are automatic, but we know now that humans can learn to some degree to control them voluntarily through behavioral therapies.

Another emergency defense controlled by the autonomic nervous system is an immobile anticipation reaction, which is also seen in animals. Sometimes when animals are frightened by a predator, they become very still to take in the sounds and observe carefully whatever is around them. In this case, there is a *decrease* in heart rate, the opposite of the fight-or-flight reaction. We also see a decrease of muscle tension and a general constriction in the blood vessels both in the skin and in the muscles. A lesser version of this occurs every time we engage in deep concentration to take in information from the world. In our ordinary functioning during any day, we go through periods where we take in information from the world in this concentrated way, and we go through periods where we anticipate a response. The autonomic nervous system mobilizes the body physiologically both to prepare for and to involve ourselves in the world.

Any situation that's stressful for us causes a response in the autonomic nervous system. When we encounter a stressful event, the activation of the autonomic nervous system causes changes from the baseline functions of heart rate, blood flow, and muscle tension. Then, when the stimulus stops, the autonomic nervous system deactivates. After a period of rest, it returns to baseline again. Anytime we encounter a new situation or something stressful, there is a pattern of activation, deactivation or rest, and return to baseline.

THE TOLL OF STRESS

When we encounter a series of stressful events, we sustain a high level of arousal without rest. This can continue for very long periods until the point of exhaustion is reached, forcing a rest. A situation of chronic stress causes a dysregulation or imbalance in the functioning of the autonomic nervous system, so that a high level of activation occurs with very little stimulus. The cells in the autonomic nervous system become hyperactive and respond with very little provocation. We start to see patterns of dysregulation in muscle tension and imbalances in the blood flow patterns. This can contribute to the development of illnesses like asthma, certain kinds of headaches, and irritable bowel syndrome, where pain and diarrhea occur without infection.

Different sorts of stress can cause these changes. There's been a lot of research on what's called life-change stress. It was found that people who had a lot of significant changes in their lives in a short time—loss through death, starting a new relationship, breaking up a relationship, suddenly coming into a lot of money, suddenly losing a lot of money, legal problems, buying a house—had an increased probability of getting sick over the next year or so.

People like routines, and routines are healthy to some degree. Too much rapid change increases the likelihood of illness. The research on life-change stress was the first research on stress in the West, but most people in their daily lives do not experience these kinds of extreme changes. Yet we all experience other kinds of stress, the daily hassles—like losing something and having to look for it, having too much to do, getting too many phone calls, waiting in traffic, having to do too many errands during the day, all the little things in life that accumulate. A poet once said that it's not the major changes in life, like people dying, that will drive one mad, it's a shoelace that breaks when there's too little time. Every time something is upsetting, it causes an activation of the autonomic nervous system. If we don't have some way of detaching, going back to a baseline of rest, then the stresses accumulate and keep the human organism in a state of high arousal. After a while this can cause health problems.

Other stressors are environmental: exposure to physical cold, pollution, noise, electromagnetic pollution. Even things like motion, flying in an airplane, can be stressful. Social stress can result from living in cities, overcrowding or too much isolation, and fighting with others. There are a variety of lifestyle stresses: poor diet, nutrition, and the use of alcohol, coffee, tobacco, and drugs. Time pressure from too many deadlines can also be stressful, as can extremes of too much and not enough exercise. People who have regular routines are usually less stressed than people who have variable routines or unpredictable schedules, such as nurses who work a different shift each day, or firefighters who never know when they'll be called to a fire.

People have begun to realize that it's not the stress that's the problem. The stress is just an event out there. Some people can be in situations that objectively are very stressful, and they show very little biological reaction. Other people produce this autonomic activation in situations that for most people are not biologically stressful. How do we explain this?

It's not just the event itself, it's how the mind interprets that event and how it copes.

There are two kinds of coping: healthy and not-so healthy. Examples of healthy coping are taking an active approach to solve the problem; or taking a different view of the problem, so it doesn't seem to be a problem any more. Another method of healthy coping involves dealing with the emotions that come up in a stressful situation by talking with or being in contact with others.

Unhealthy coping includes repressing or denying the problem, or just wishing the problem would go away, fantasizing about a more pleasant state. Instead of dealing with the problem, one is constantly preoccupied with getting away from it. The problem doesn't go away, and even though the mind goes elsewhere, the body still has a reaction.

Other examples of unhealthy coping with emotions are blaming and numbing. Blaming is a form of self-hatred characteristic of Westerners. Numbing is when people lose their ability to be aware of feelings as a result of extreme psychological trauma such as abuse.

Trauma and Its Toll

We have studied people who have survived various kinds of psychological trauma: people who have been sexually abused as children, victims of crime, and survivors of war, including those who have been wounded or had near-death experiences, people who were imprisoned and systematically tortured for political reasons, and also refugees. Most of my experience with refugees has been with Central Americans, but we also have worked with refugees from South Asia, primarily from Cambodia and to some extent from Vietnam. I imagine you must face similar problems with your own people who have been tortured or have left their homeland.

When we work with these individuals, it's very hard to start with psychological treatment. Instead we start with environmental interventions, because if people are refugees, often their culture has been fragmented. The first level of intervention is to help them reestablish their community, and to meet basic needs like housing and food. When they come to a foreign country, they don't know how to manage or how to go about getting help, so we provide them with assistance in establishing community. The work is made more difficult by the fact that American policy in accepting people from other countries has been to distribute them in different cities around the country. This is not a good approach, because what people really need is to reconstruct their sense of community. If survivors are scattered in different communities, they feel very isolated. They don't know the language and they don't have contact with people from their own culture. So, to the extent that it's possible, we try to encourage people to live within the same community. We also teach basics, such as enough English for them to manage daily life, but the priority is always reestablishing the sense of relationship in community.

The community is not simply the community of people, but also the practices of their culture, so we particularly encourage people to reconstruct their arts and crafts, and to participate in their religion. For example, with the Cambodians in the Boston area, we would encourage them to go to the Buddhist temple. For the Cambodians, it is especially difficult in that only the poor farmers survived the Cambodian holocaust; most of the professional people were killed and all the institutions of the culture, including schools and religious institutions, were destroyed.

I was very impressed when I went to the Tibetan Children's Village that people there are trying to do exactly the same thing as the researchers in the West have recommended for the first stage of treatment for victims of torture and severe holocaust experiences: to get the survivors to live in a community with their own people and provide them with basic needs, food and shelter. The next step is to get them to participate in their own cultural heritage. It's not enough for the refugees who come from Tibet to simply live in the community; they should practice Dharma and get involved in the arts.

If you try to provide people with psychological treatment at this point, it doesn't work. Even though they may have nightmares every night, and they may be very anxious and agitated, there's very little you can do until you first connect them to the community. That first level of intervention may take a few years, and unfortunately they have to live with the extreme pain and despair until they get connected. Sometimes medication helps, but it's complicated because they may not understand the medication or want to take it. We try to provide them with the same medications they would get in their own culture, but generally we don't treat the effects of the torture directly at first.

Once they are connected to their own community and can speak enough English to get by or at least work with translators, the next level is to work psychologically. We do this both individually and in groups. Some people won't work in groups because of the cultural background. The refugees from Central America include both the extreme left and members of the death squads on the extreme right who left because of human rights pressure. Both sides live in the same community, so the war continues. They won't come together in groups because they're afraid the person next to them is an enemy. It's easier to work with other groups like Cambodians who will meet together in groups because that group connection is very healthy for them. You'll probably find this true also for the Tibetans. In the groups, we get them to talk about everyday things. We don't have them talk about their experiences of torture in the group because it stirs them up and makes their symptoms much worse, both physical and mental.

The next stage of the treatment is to work with them individually in a process similar to psychotherapy. Many refugees don't understand this, but it can be developed in terms of their own culture. Many people who have suffered the extreme violation of systematic torture have great difficulty in feeling safe with any other person or even when they're alone.

They're always afraid that someone will come to harm them. They relive their experience many times over in their dreams, and in their waking state they have flashbacks or intrusive memories of the trauma, which are very difficult to cope with. We have them do visualizations around the theme of safety. We ask them if they've ever had the experience of safety in their lives, and then we have them imagine themselves in that situation so they can learn to generate the feeling of safety at will. If they say they've never felt safe in their lives, we ask them to imagine how other people might feel safe and then to visualize themselves in that situation.

These visualizations of safety last anywhere from ten minutes to an hour. When they try to visualize, there is often a shift and memories of the torture start coming up. At that point we tell them to switch to visualizing another safe place. If the intrusive memories come up again, we ask them to switch again, so they learn the skill of controlling the very arising of memories in their mind. If they have been systematically tortured, they may need to spend as long as three years doing only the visualizations of safety, but eventually they feel safe and confident. Because of this emphasis, safety becomes the foundation of the therapy relationship. Once they become more confident about controlling their own state of mind in this way, we introduce other visualizations. Eventually they'll start to remember the torture experiences in bits and pieces, and they will start to talk about it. We try to have them talk about it only a little bit at a time. Eventually they'll be able to talk more easily and make sense of it. Things will settle down and they'll go on to lead a normal life. So that's roughly the sequence that we follow: first, environmental interventions, reestablishing the community and the sense of connection to the culture; then work in groups and the visualizations around safety; and finally the actual memory integration.

DALAI LAMA: Among the Tibetan refugees who spent long times in concentration camps in Tibet, there have been some who reported their time in prison was very valuable, because they found their spiritual practice went the very best in prison. Generally speaking, it's quite rare among Tibetans that these traumatic experiences have left deep scars in the mind. If experts in this field were to interview the refugees from Tibet, I think they would find some relative differences from their other findings.

DANIEL GOLEMAN: Your Holiness, do they not have the nightmares that are so typical of torture victims in other places?

DALAI LAMA: Some may well have nightmares. When I was in Lhasa with the Chinese Communists all around, I had nightmares as well. Even today, thirty years later, I still occasionally have them. [*laughs*] But there's no anxiety or fear involved.

There are a very large number of newcomers from Tibet, from their teens up to the age of thirty or so, and many of them have spent their lives in concentration camps and prisons. These are monks who are now studying in the monastic universities in South India. Among them, it's very rare to find any who have had the symptoms typical of posttraumatic stress disorder. In fact, these students turn out to be better scholars than those who were raised in India.

DANIEL GOLEMAN: Is that because of what you explained earlier about the practice of seeing one's own suffering as a spiritual opportunity? Is that what they're doing during the torture?

DALAI LAMA: Yes.

JON KABAT-ZINN: It would be very interesting to study the Tibetans who have been incarcerated and tortured.

DANIEL BROWN: There have been studies of people who survived the Nazi concentration camps and of prisoners of war who were in the "tiger cages" in South Asia. The people who best survived those experiences had very strong religious or philosophical belief systems that protected them from what would be the expected results of torture.

DALAI LAMA: But I think the majority of the Cambodians and Vietnamese are also Buddhists.

DANIEL BROWN: There are three types of reactions to torture experiences, or to any kind of trauma, for that matter. First are intrusive experiences like bad memories and nightmares. The second are what we call numbing experiences, not feeling anything. The third is a kind of physiological reactivity. The autonomic nervous system is altered, and a high level of arousal continues. This physiological reactivity can exist even among people who have strong belief systems. Based on the research that has been done in the West, I would expect that if we measured your monks physiologically they might still show signs of this, although they may not complain of nightmares.

DALAI LAMA: It should be checked. It's easy to do. At Sera Monastery there are about 1,000 of these youngsters, at Drepung Loseling about 500 or 600, and at Ganden about 250 or 300. In my experience with these students over many years, I've never seen any abnormal cases. They're just like any other young monks.

DANIEL BROWN: What you're describing is very rare.

FRANCISCO VARELA: I personally know several of my compatriots from Chile who were tortured by Pinochet's secret police after the military coup that toppled the democratic government of Salvador Allende. There is not a single one who hasn't had some or all of the symptoms, the nightmares and physiological disruptions. These, of course, are not Buddhists.

DALAI LAMA: Are there differences among your people between those who have strong religious beliefs and others?

FRANCISCO VARELA: The people who were persecuted and tortured were all from the left, so if they had a strong belief system it was likely to be political. They might have had some Christian values because they were brought up in that culture.

DANIEL BROWN: It's also true that they were being tortured by people who had the same religious background as themselves.

FRANCISCO VARELA: They were tortured in a civilian war, by people from their own country.

DANIEL BROWN: Whereas the Chinese are not Buddhist. There's a vast difference in being tortured by an enemy who's not part of your own people.

FRANCISCO VARELA: Maybe.

DALAI LAMA: When Tibetans describe their experiences in prison, they point out that the reason they were in prison was not because they did something illegal or wrong, like killing or stealing, but because they were freedom fighters acting on their principles.

FRANCISCO VARELA: Yes, but Chileans have the same feelings too.

DALAI LAMA: So this should be the same. Does that kind of attitude help?

FRANCISCO VARELA: Yes, it does help. But out of the several I know, only a few were able to pull their lives together again based on that strong feeling. The majority of them were broken in one way or another: their families broke up, they couldn't continue to work, they had insomnia, they had cancer. Even with this righteous feeling, somewhere there was always an ambivalence, a weakening of that strength, a feeling that maybe what we thought was right wasn't. Maybe for the Tibetans the sense of principle is much stronger.

JON KABAT-ZINN: Your Holiness, you said yesterday that in the Buddhist view, evil is ignorance, and therefore a Buddhist might feel compassion for the ignorance even if it meant great pain for oneself. I read the very moving account of your own physician, a Tibetan doctor who was tortured for years in a Chinese prison. He said that he never got angry at these people even though they were torturing him, but continued to maintain a sense of compassion for their profound ignorance that they could do such things to people. The American psychiatrist who interviewed this man said he was astounded that he could come out of that experience and show no signs of posttraumatic stress syndrome from a clinical Western psychiatric perspective. He was not bitter; he showed no ill will; he didn't have physical or psychological problems associated with it. Do you believe that this is common among the vast majority of monks who have been coming out of Tibet after being in prison?

DALAI LAMA: It's very difficult to say, because some of these monks are very strong in their feeling of bitterness toward the Chinese.

DANIEL GOLEMAN: So they're not feeling compassion for the torturer.

DALAI LAMA: It seems not. [*laughs*]

DANIEL GOLEMAN: Then, Your Holiness, what were they doing other than practicing compassion that made the difference so that they didn't have these problems?

DALAI LAMA: One factor is their belief in karma. They attribute their suffering to mistakes they have made in past lives. This is a very common conviction among Tibetans.

DANIEL GOLEMAN: That alone? Was there something more?

DALAI LAMA: Taking refuge is an important factor, and this is common to all religions. Thinking about the disadvantages of *samsara*, the cycle of existence, and reflecting on impermanence could be other factors. Finally, there is a very strong conviction that truth will finally win out.

DANIEL BROWN: Your Holiness, in the diagnostic statistical manual that is our authoritative text on diagnosis of psychiatric conditions in the West, they define trauma as an event that's extraordinary and unusual enough that it will produce symptoms in almost everyone. It's defined that way because in the West, it's very rare to see somebody who doesn't have these symptoms after torture. If what you are saying is true, we have a lot to learn from your people about how they protect themselves from the symptoms of posttraumatic stress that are experienced by almost everyone else in this kind of situation. This information is extraordinary to us.

PART THREE

Skillful Means and Medicine

6

Mindfulness as Medicine

SHARON SALZBERG AND
JON KABAT-ZINN

SHARON SALZBERG'S overview of the Theravadin tradition of meditation serves as a basis for the description of mindfulness practice taught by Jon Kabat-Zinn at the Stress Reduction Clinic at the University of Massachusetts Medical Center in Worcester, Massachusetts. Such medical uses of mindfulness meditation are becoming increasingly popular in Western medical settings.

Stripped of its religious context, mindfulness meditation is simply learning to have an open accepting attitude toward whatever arises in one's mind, while watching the movements of the mind. This very simplicity makes it useful as a stress reduction technique.

Jon Kabat-Zinn explains how mindfulness meditation has been incorporated into his stress reduction and relaxation clinic. Although meditation techniques have a long history of use in the context of spiritual training, it is only recently in the West that these methods have begun to be systematically applied and studied as part of a medical and psychological treatment regime.

Jon Kabat-Zinn's presentation synthesizes much of what

has been discussed so far. He has attempted to bring some techniques of Buddhist meditation into the mainstream culture of the West. Since mindfulness meditation is not presented in a spiritual context, Kabat-Zinn believes it can address some of the needs of people who are suffering throughout the world, but for one reason or another are not interested in Buddhism or any other belief system.

MINDFULNESS IN THERAVADIN BUDDHISM

SHARON SALZBERG: When we teach mindfulness meditation, usually we have people begin by just sitting quietly and feeling the breath at one location in the body, some place where it's very clear to them, such as the rising and falling of the abdomen. We ask them to simply feel the breath at first, and then to observe anything that becomes predominant in their awareness. Thus they become aware of many different objects at different times: sounds, images, or sensations in the body. We ask them to try to observe this experience very directly, very clearly, in a straightforward way without getting lost in interpretation or judgment about what is happening. For example, if somebody has physical pain, rather than thinking, "This is good," or "This is bad," or "I'm a bad person because I have pain," we suggest they should very clearly note the sensation of heat, or pressure, or tension, so they can see how the sensations change constantly and that there's nothing solid or permanent about "the pain." Also, they come to recognize that they do not control what sensations arise in the body. The pain did not arise in response to their desire, so they do not have to feel they own it. It doesn't belong to them, it is only the coming together of conditions to create a sensation. We ask them to observe very deeply so they really see the arising phenomenon break apart even as they're observing it, and in that way they can see into the nature of their experience. If they can do that, then the mind becomes very still and very calm. The mind is not running to the past and to the future, but instead has a quality of stability and stillness, and actually rests in the experience of the moment.

We also emphasize a purity of observation. Whether the object is the breath, or the pain, or whatever else arises, they observe it without grasping, aversion, or ignorance. Whether it's pleasant or painful or neutral, the object of the meditation should not lead the mind to develop more grasping, or aversion, or ignorance. We try to make a distinction between mindfulness that is just ordinary attention, and mindfulness that has this quality of purity. We teach people to practice continuously, whether they are sitting, walking, drinking a cup of tea, or doing work in the world. We may focus on the breath to begin with, but the practice eventually becomes all inclusive. Whatever activity we do becomes meditation practice.

DALAI LAMA: You don't add any special analysis or investigation to the mindfulness?

SHARON SALZBERG: No, we've seen that pure awareness brings understanding and insight without analysis. Particularly when there is strong continuity of mindfulness and people are able to practice regularly, they come to see a thought as just a thought, for example. They do not feel governed or driven by any particular thought that comes up in the mind, but instead can let go of whatever it is.

DALAI LAMA: When you identify something as merely a thought, what comes to your mind? How do you identify it? What is this "mere thought"?

SHARON SALZBERG: Our awareness makes a transition so that the content or subject of the thought is not so important. What we are observing is the process of thinking. When we see that a thought is not solid, that it has no substance, and the actual meaning of the thought does not necessarily effect an association or reaction, it's as if we have observed the very nature of change. If someone then has the thought "I am a very sick person," the fact of the thought's content does not seem so striking. The mind intuitively recognizes the nature of thought, that it simply comes and goes. With this particular approach, we don't try to change a bad thought to a good thought, but rather to see the nature of thought itself.

DALAI LAMA: Once again it raises the question, what do you recognize as the nature of thought?

SHARON SALZBERG: The object at that moment is actually change. In seeing this experience of thinking, the mind is lighting upon the fact that all arising phenomena are fleeting and transitory.

DALAI LAMA: This fleeting character, of course, is something that is true of all conditioned phenomena. What is the unique nature of thought that distinguishes it from other phenomena that are also fleeting? I ask this because there are many types of meditation that are concerned with the very nature of the mind itself. In doing something like this, we speak of gaining direct insight into various things, including thought. You see then that the thought is mere thought. I'm wondering what fresh insights you have as a result of this technique, when you gain this possibly unprecedented insight into the nature of mere thought. How do you now perceive thought in a way different from ordinary perception of thought?

SHARON SALZBERG: The insight or the understanding is of emptiness. It is also one of interdependence between all things. We see that the mind and body are in constant relationship, with a continual chain of cause and effect between body and mind being who we truly are. The reason I emphasize the thinking process is because, as much as we tend to identify with the body and be attached to it, there is so much more attachment and identification with the mind. To borrow an image from the Tibetan tradition, the insightful mind sees thoughts as clouds moving through the sky, not owning them, not controlling them. For people like Jon's patients, even a little insight into the empty, insubstantial nature of thought provides a very great feeling of freedom.

DALAI LAMA: Would you explain what you mean by empty in this context?

SHARON SALZBERG: Insubstantial, without a core.

DALAI LAMA: Anatman.[1]

SHARON SALZBERG: Yes.

DALAI LAMA: So the emptiness or absence of identity that you are referring to would be one of the three marks of existence [i.e., emptiness, unsatisfactoriness, impermanence].[2]

SHARON SALZBERG: Yes.

DALAI LAMA: Very good.

SHARON SALZBERG: This kind of practice is powerful because people can do it without any belief system or religious feeling. Yet, we try to introduce it with a very strong moral base. From that base they can have the awareness that experiences calm, clarity, sensitivity, and an understanding about themselves and about their lives.

DALAI LAMA: How much meditation is done by average practitioners following this technique, or by those who have found some real benefit in the practice? How many sessions do they do each day, and what is the duration of each session? Also, how long is it before they find some manifest benefit? A week, a month, a year?

SHARON SALZBERG: Usually, people sit in meditation about one hour a day, if they can. To some extent they benefit immediately or they would not keep doing it. It's not as though they come with faith to begin with; they need a good experience to have any kind of confidence. Usually, I think it takes several months before people feel established and confident in the practice.

DALAI LAMA: What is the distinction between the *samatha* and *vipassana* practice?

SHARON SALZBERG: In the *samatha* practice we choose a single object such as the breath or a mantra and focus on that alone, whereas in *vipassana* we open up our awareness to observe all experience without a specific object. Rather than emphasizing union or oneness with a specific object, *vipassana* emphasizes the changing nature of things, to see the three marks of existence in every experience.

DALAI LAMA: Very good. Is the training that you give to these meditators extracted from the meditative techniques of the Sri Lankan and Burmese traditions? Is it a combination of different traditions, or is it specific to one particular tradition?

SHARON SALZBERG: It's particular to one lineage of the Burmese tradition.

DALAI LAMA: Very good. Do you have a basis for this practice in the Sutras?

SHARON SALZBERG: The *Satipatthana-sutra*. Your Holiness, Lee Yearley quoted the philosopher William James, who said that a religion has to keep growing like a plant grows or else it will die, and yet at the same time it needs to maintain and protect its essential tradition. This is the problem: to both grow and maintain what is most essential. Could you speak about what seems most essential to preserve in Buddhist teaching and in what ways it might actually be able to change and grow?

DALAI LAMA: I believe that the essence is compassion and the wisdom that realizes emptiness. These both pertain to the basic reality with which they're confronted; they pertain to the path, as method and wisdom; and they also pertain to the fruition of the path. Each of these has this dual aspect of compassion and wisdom. How Buddhadharma should grow, I'm not sure. I think in all the major religions, the basic system does not need to change, but change does need to take place in the cultural aspect or social habits. We see an evolution from Tibetan Buddhism to Western Buddhism, including

American Buddhism. Just as Tibetan Buddhism naturally evolved, so, I suspect, there will naturally evolve a Western Buddhism, and an American Buddhism. This is something that has to be developed gradually.

THE CLINICAL USES OF MINDFULNESS

JON KABAT-ZINN: Let me attempt to take into a larger domain something that the Buddhist meditative perspective can offer to the West. It may address some of the very deep and severe needs of people who are suffering throughout the world, but for one reason or another are not interested in Buddhism or any other belief system. They are not interested in enlightenment, but they are very interested in the relief of suffering, in particular their own suffering. The question arises: Is there some wisdom unique to Buddhism that would not be distorted or damaged by making it available to people who are suffering? Could this help them become more whole as human beings, less fragmented, and less contributing to their own continual suffering?

My own training, meager as it is, is in the Theravadin and Zen traditions. The program I will describe reflects a range of different meditative techniques that I personally have tried to introduce into a mainstream Western medical setting. In this context, if I came in with my head shaved, wearing robes and beads, and chanting in Tibetan or Sanskrit or Korean, it would not go over very well with most people, no matter how good the teaching was. That would not be the most effective or skillful way to introduce whatever wisdom or essence of the practice might be accessible. Nowadays people know about meditation but they have a very incomplete view of it. We want to teach people that meditation is not making your mind blank, but instead is learning to see things as they are and to live with things as they are.

One of the values of Buddhist meditation that we know very little about in mainstream daily life in the West is the quality of stillness. You may have observed that we run around a lot in the West. Americans have developed this to a fine art. We are constantly engaged in doing, then we fall into bed exhausted, wake up the next day, and start more doing, more running. It doesn't require too much depth of perception in oneself to notice that often we don't know who's doing the doing. Very often we feel cut off from our own experience and feelings. We are driven by the mind, by thought, by expectations, by fear, by wanting to get somewhere else. If you always want to be some place else, then you are never actually where you are, and therefore not fully alive. Nor are you capable of dealing with the pressures and difficulties that arise if your mind is inattentive and is half not here. In stressful or threatening situations, your reactions will be highly conditioned and automatic. The deeper levels of intelligence and wisdom that come from clear and full seeing will not be available to you because of this foggy cloud in the mind.

This is also true of the body. As we discussed earlier, many people are not sensitive to their body on a deep level until something goes wrong. Then they get very upset and run to an expert who's supposed to make it all better, but often cannot. Although Western medicine has developed remarkable technological advances in the past twenty years, much of it is diagnostic. It tells you what the problem is, but doesn't necessarily fix it. There are very few cures in Western medicine.

We thought that it would be wonderful to set up a clinic based on mindfulness training within a Western medical center, because a hospital is really a magnet for suffering. It seemed a skillful way to introduce notions of stillness, clear seeing, mindfulness, and the shift from running around all the time to a more inwardly focused being. If we could offer patients something as a complement to their medical treatment, perhaps they would grow and heal in a way that the medical treatment by itself doesn't provide. The program may also help patients comply with the medical treatment, which is more difficult when the mind is agitated and wants things to be different from the way they are.

Let me take you on a brief tour of the principles and structure of our clinic, the Stress Reduction and Relaxation Program at the University of Massachusetts Medical Center in Worcester, and how we work with meditation. Then I will show you some results of the clinic for a variety of serious medical conditions, and their implications not only for physical symptoms but also mental changes that may reflect human growth or development. I will finish with how we have been trying to integrate these principles of mindfulness, clear seeing, and nondoing into many aspects of the hospital's work, not just for patients but also in training doctors and medical students. We are training them to be more sensitive and observant, and changing the ways they work with their patients.

A famous doctor said the most important thing about patient care is caring for the patient, but very often in big hospitals, the patient gets lost and falls through the cracks in the system, especially with chronic diseases. This clinic provides a safety net to catch these people and offer them one more chance before they fall through. That chance is an opportunity to explore on a deep level how they might help themselves. They have sought help from other people in all sorts of places, but we ask, "Have you considered the inner resources, perhaps even the wisdom, that already exists in your body and mind? If you can uncover it and develop a way to use that energy, then perhaps, together with your doctors, you can move toward greater levels of health and healing." This is not curing, but healing. A cure just magically makes it all better somehow, but healing transforms both body and mind on a deep level. One sees differently and comes to terms with one's illness. Even missing an arm and a leg you could still be a whole, complete human being, fully alive on the most fundamental level. This is not easy to achieve, but it is possible. A human being could perceive that wholeness, completeness, and health are not necessarily dependent on two arms and two legs or even being free from cancer or AIDS. We feel very strongly that as long as you are alive and breathing, there is more right with you than wrong. We challenge people to focus on what is right with them and let the doctors take care of what's wrong.

In the *Satipatthana-sutra*, the Buddha gives one of his simple but extremely profound messages: that the true path does not have to be elaborate, that there is power in simplicity, and that mindfulness is a cornerstone of meditative practice. Our point of departure for the clinic is that mindfulness is very powerfully healing for suffering of all kinds. The hypothesis is that mindfulness can heal whether one is operating within a Buddhist context or not. Can we demonstrate this in a non-Buddhist, mainstream medical setting?

The clinic is located at the University of Massachusetts Medical Center (UMMC), a large medical school and hospital. The center has 400 beds for inpatients and sees thousands of outpatients every day. It's a very young medical school, started in 1970, which may explain why I have been able to do this work there. As institutions grow, they develop "arthritis" and "hardening of the attitudes" and are much less open to new ideas. UMMC is also a major trauma center where patients are flown in by helicopter from a very large area. The suffering in this hospital isn't all on the part of the patients, either. The staff members have a great deal of stress.

Stress has become a way of life for most Americans. That would not necessarily be bad. It's not so much the stress that's the problem, it's how you cope with it. This depends on how you see it, and how you see it depends partly on *whether* you see it. A lot of people do not see or feel the stress, as a fish swimming in water doesn't see the water. We are unconscious of much of the stress in our lives and we live very mechanically, on automatic pilot. The mind is constantly agitated and is very often either in the past with memories or in the future, but rarely in the present.

We have been using the term *stress* a lot here, but no one has defined it. I like the word because it is so broad that it includes all types of suffering. No one knows what a stress reduction clinic means, but everybody wants to come. From a scientific point of view, the word *stress* is awkward because it indicates both the stimulus that causes a problem and the response—the problem itself. One definition is that stress is the response of the organism to the entire range of pressure and demands that are placed on it to adapt. So anything can be stressful, but it doesn't have to be. It depends on whether there's pressure to change. Change itself is stressful, of course, because it means that you have to adapt. An animal living where there is suddenly no more food will either die or will have to migrate to find food. Moving is the adaptation that enables the animal to continue living. Many of our stresses are mental, but they still require us to change or adapt. A death in the family is a big stress, because there's enormous loss, and then one has to adapt in some way by coming to terms with the loss. If one does not adapt, then the organism somehow falls out of harmony. Even on the level of the nervous system and the immune system, there can be dysregulation after a death in the family. However, after a while one recovers, time heals all wounds, and one returns to inner balance. If one has many stresses in one's life, one can reach the point where there is continuous anxiety, and health breaks down.

THE STRESS REDUCTION AND RELAXATION PROGRAM

The Stress Reduction and Relaxation Program takes the form of a course. If you want someone to change his or her life, you can't just say, "You've been working too hard; you need to change your life; just relax." If people knew how to relax, they wouldn't have come to the doctor in the first place. One has to teach: to encounter the person on a deep level and give him or her enough time to grow and experiment, and to come back and ask questions. We thought the best way to do this would be a course. The training in mindfulness would be its foundation and would unify the practices. As Sharon mentioned, no matter how skillful you become in mindfulness and in developing calmness and stillness and relaxation, if it does not spill over into daily life, there's no wisdom. It's no use sitting like a Buddha for one hour if the rest of the time you're out of control like a bull. You can get very deluded that you are a great meditator without any awareness of serious problems with your work or family. We believe that mindfulness in daily life is extremely important to the essence of meditation training.

The context of the course is how to take better care of yourself, how to live more skillfully and fully, and how to move, if possible, toward greater health and well-being. It is not a replacement for medical treatment, but a complement to it. It's important that our clinic is in the department of medicine, rather than in the psychiatry department. Very often when people have problems with stress, the doctor finds nothing medically wrong and refers them to a psychiatrist. The implication is that there's something wrong with the mind. In the West, of course, the mind is separated from the body and is treated in a different department on the eighth floor of the hospital. Many people do not respond well to this approach. They perceive the pain in the body and not in the mind, and they don't want to be identified as crazy. Placing the clinic in the department of medicine communicates that the nondualistic view of mind and body is an essential part of what Western medicine and science is growing to become. Of course, for convenience' sake, we speak about the mind and the body, and there are very important differences. However, if we don't understand that at a deep level they are also the same, it creates problems. In one pan of the balance is a very powerful, very beautiful technological medicine, with its X-rays, CAT scans, surgery, drugs, and all. On the other side, is behavioral, or mind/body, medicine, the power of the mind, and what a person can do for himself or herself. For medicine to maintain balance, the more money that goes into technological medicine, the more energy really needs to go into the other side.

In our clinic, we use an approach that is very different from the medical and psychiatric models, and also from the model of Buddhist teaching. In medicine or psychiatry, the first step

is to diagnose the problem and then to
ment. Likewise, when a person asks a
lem in meditation, the answer addres
and is not the same for everyone.
stress reduction clinic, we have set up a v
regarding general versus specific interventions.
neric training with large groups of people and focus
their individual problems, but on what they have in commo.
that's already right. They all have different diseases, their
own family troubles, their own genetics, their own work situation, and their own doctor who takes care of the specifics of
the medical treatment. We teach them all the same thing: how
to pay attention—in other words, how to be mindful, how to
tune in.

We do give our patients some individual attention and
modify the instructions to their specific needs and circumstances. It's not as if this is a factory and we don't care what
their problems are; it's more that we want to address what
they have in common. We do an evaluation interview one-
on-one with each patient who is referred to the clinic, to evaluate them before and after the training, as well as doing long-
term follow-up. In the interview, we want to hear patients'
stories, who they are and how they truly feel about their illnesses and their bodies. We try to really listen to the person
and experience his or her situation with some compassion.
Then we tell the person what to expect. Most patients don't
understand what it means when we say we'll do meditation
or mindful yoga, but they can choose to enroll or not. Ninety
percent of the people referred do enroll.

The course is eight weeks long, and patients come once a
week for two and a half hours. There are thirty people in the
class, sitting in a circle. They also have homework, consisting
of forty-five minutes of meditation practice per day, six days
a week. We give them one day off for good behavior. We
don't just tell people to go home and practice what we taught
them in class, but instead we give them audiotapes to guide
them. For homework, they repeat one side of the tape over
and over. We tell them they don't have to like it, they just

to do it. They also do some awareness exercises in a kbook, writing down thoughts and feelings.

Taking forty-five minutes a day to do nothing is a big life-style change. The Buddhist tradition honors that as what is obviously necessary to move toward wholeness and reduce fragmentation, but in the West it's not obvious at all. It's almost anti-American to propose that someone take forty-five minutes and just be. These people are there because their doctor has told them they need to learn to deal with stress, not for enlightenment or to practice meditation or yoga. They're willing to do it because we explain it to them as an adventure: that perhaps there is something new to learn here, some new source of vitality.

In the sixth week of the course, we have a silent meditation retreat for eight hours. We work with about 150 people at a time, and we run the meditation retreat in silence for all of these people together. Four people teach the program, guiding the participants through a whole day of mindfulness in sitting, walking, eating, all in silence with no eye contact. This is very unusual for Westerners, especially if they have not been exposed to meditation. For many people, it's the first time in their lives they've been awake but silent for eight hours.

THE MINDFUL ATTITUDE: BEGINNER'S MIND

Certain aspects of mindfulness training are very important in the clinic: nonjudgment, patience, acceptance, and trust. Also important are nonstriving, letting go, and what is known as beginner's mind.

We don't teach the principles of nonjudgment, patience, acceptance, and trust as directives, as they are taught in the sutras. Instead, we try to introduce them naturally and coherently in our discussion of the homework and meditation practice each week. The discussion is pretty explicit, however. We talk a lot about nonjudgmental self-observation. For example, when we have a discussion after the first week of meditation practice, some people have had a deep experience of relaxation and are very excited about it, while others have only experienced tension and pain, or have fallen asleep every time they've tried to meditate. When they start to judge themselves and feel that they are no good at this, we remind them that their job is just to watch, to see clearly, and not to judge. Also, we remind them to be patient: "Just because one person had an experience in the first week doesn't mean you have to proceed at the same pace. Just take it moment by moment."

In this way, we introduce acceptance and trust—not trust in me, or the Dalai Lama, or any external authority, but trust in one's own inner being. This is primary, because in a religious context we are often quick to make someone else the hero and to reduce ourselves. It's very important that people take responsibility for their own lives and not simply accept authority in a way that reduces their own creativity and power.

Nonstriving is another very big part of the mindfulness practice. This is again very anti-American, not to push to get someplace. It comes up because everybody is referred with a problem. We have thirty people in the room and each one has a problem. She wants to lower her blood pressure; he wants to reduce his headaches; another has AIDS and wants to deal with the fact of his approaching death or his family who has disowned him. Everybody has so much pain, emotional as well as physical. We say explicitly, right at the beginning, "Now that you've come with your problem, we want you to suspend judgment. For the next eight weeks, don't try to make your problem go away. Don't try to do anything. Just do the homework and see what happens. At the end of the program you can tell us whether this was of some benefit or not, but we're not going to try to lower the blood pressure or push the pain out of our bodies. No striving." One way we express this is, "We're going to teach you how to be so relaxed that it's okay to be tense."

We also try to give people a sense of what is sometimes called beginner's mind, the notion that every moment is new.

It's a bad idea to think that because you've been meditating for a long time you've reached someplace. Both the "you" and the "someplace" become problems. It's important to maintain a sense of freshness and not to think, "I've seen this all before," or "I've been doing this for three weeks and I know what meditation is now." Whether you've had good, bad, or neutral experiences, do not project them into the future and think, "Because I had a good meditation today, I will have a good meditation tomorrow." This whole notion of being in the present moment is extremely new for most people in the West. I might add that it's most difficult for intellectuals and scholars, people who do a lot of thinking for a living.

Another aspect is letting go, the capacity to see clearly and just not touch. We distinguish between letting go and pushing away. Letting go is letting things be, nonattachment.

I think these qualities—letting go, beginner's mind, non-striving, and nonjudgment—lead to a certain kind of wisdom if they are practiced to any extent. One can be attached without knowing it; mindfulness allows you see the attachment. Even if you don't let go of it, the awareness of the attachment is already greater wisdom than there was before.

Other qualities that we don't teach explicitly are embedded in the way we try to include what we teach in our own lives: generosity, compassion, and sympathetic joy. Rather than talking about compassion, which in the West sometimes sounds very stilted, we try to let these qualities come through our own being in our interactions. When someone in the class goes through a crisis, or is crying, or whatever, there are many different ways to respond with compassion. At those times, if one can come from one's own heart, rather than from the head, that is a sign of a skillful teacher. Many of these qualities are best taught by embodying them in yourself. In the medical system in the West, this is not well understood. Instead techniques are found, and then applied to people when the need arises, like a pill or an injection. It's not understood that a psychotherapist who teaches relaxation or meditation needs to practice himself. After all, there's nothing wrong with the doctor or therapist. It's the patient who has the problem or has to take the medicine. This orientation is very different from the model we use. We would not consider hiring somebody in our clinic who had not been meditating for years in some tradition, with intensive periods of practice such as retreats. However, you could find many people who have been practicing for years who would not be able to teach in this way, for many reasons. It's not easy to find people who are qualified to teach this.

I mentioned that a large part of this is really training in how to move from doing to nondoing, and to develop a certain degree of calmness and stability in one's own mind. We often use the image that the mind is like the surface of water. When strong winds blow, it can be very choppy. People think, wrongly, that they have to force the choppiness to go away, as if they will become calm by putting a big glass plate on top of the waves. But you can just go down ten or twenty feet beneath the waves and let the choppiness remain where it is. By observing the choppiness, you can learn to contact the sense of calm that's always there within yourself. You don't have to make it happen, it's already present. The skill lies in learning how to contact it in oneself. The spirit of the practice is not making it a goal.

This is all an elaborate way of saying that meditation is wrongly thought of in the United States as a technique, or a lot of techniques. My understanding is that meditation in a larger sense is really a way of being, an ability to generalize the quality of mindfulness. Rather than performing some kind of manipulation of one's attention at certain times, you develop a continuity of awareness that allows all of your life to become an expression of your meditation practice. Whether something expected or unexpected happens, good or bad, one can bring to it the same quality of awareness, dispassionate nonattachment, and clear seeing. It's not something that you do; it's a nondoing.

Meditation Techniques

Now that I've said that meditation is not techniques, I will tell you about the three major formal techniques we teach. All of them use the breath as the central object of awareness, the foundation where one starts at the level of the body.

One of the three techniques is the body scan. Because many people come to us with back pain, and many are older, in wheelchairs, or on crutches, we don't ask them to sit in the full lotus posture. They would not come back for the next class. It would also create the wrong understanding that the only way to meditate is in the lotus posture. So we have people lie down, if possible on their backs. We ask them to get in touch with their breathing and keep their awareness on the breath, starting at the belly. At a certain point they move their awareness into the toes of the left foot. They just try to bring their attention into this region of the body and then connect it with their breathing. As they breathe in, they start at the nose and follow the breath as best they can in the mind, down into the toes. Then they follow it back up. As they move up, there is a sense that the body is erased, becoming much more transparent. Each time they breathe out, they let go of any tension in that region. If it flows out, fine; if it doesn't flow out, it's also fine. They feel the sensations, focus on them, and breathe with the sensations. If the sensations are strong they note that they're strong; if they're weak they note that they're weak. If they are neutral, or can't be found, then they note that they can't find them. In other words, if there's no feeling there, they tune into not feeling. They can't go wrong.

Then, they move their awareness up the left leg and gradually through the entire body, deep as well as on the surface. It's a long trip. It takes about forty-five minutes, and in each moment they are seeing and letting go, seeing and letting go, over and over again. They do this six days a week for two weeks, for forty-five minutes each day.

All these people have serious medical problems, and they have strong emotions about the parts of their bodies that are not well. As they do the body scan, they learn to accept the bare experience of each part, including the area of the problem. They learn to accept the experience of it in the moment, and let go of it as they move on into another region. Many people have never had a deep experience of being comfortable inside their own body since they were children. One of the first things that happens, of course, is that people get very relaxed and fall asleep. Many don't get further than the left toe, or maybe the knee. Once they learn not to fall asleep, but to remain with full awareness and an appreciation of the body, they often report deep experiences of relaxation that they have never had before. That's one reason we use the body scan. It's very busy because you're always doing something; it keeps the mind busy.

DALAI LAMA: There is a parallel practice in the *Guh-yasamaja-tantra* which is called the Vajra recitation. The difference is that that practice entails visualizing the channels, whereas in the practice you describe there is no visualization. It is said that with the Vajra Recitation, advanced meditators can also cure certain illnesses, such as problems with their eyes.

JON KABAT-ZINN: I think we would all be very interested in hearing more about this practice.

DALAI LAMA: But to practice it you have to receive initiation. [laughter]

JON KABAT-ZINN: After the body scan the next technique we introduce is sitting meditation.

When people begin with the awareness of breathing, they first discover that it's not so easy to pay attention to the breath. It comes as a shock, but it is also a very important and positive discovery for ordinary people to realize that the mind has a life of its own. The mind does not necessarily stay on the breath just because the person decides it should. Once they begin to feel comfortable with riding the waves of the breath, nonjudgmentally, moment by moment, then we expand the field of awareness to include the entire body, not scanning but just being aware of the body as a whole. If there is very strong sensation of pain, or stored emotional pain, in a particular region, they can choose to focus on that. If there's no region that predominates or demands attention, then they focus on the experience of the body as a whole and also, if possible, a sense of it as being complete—that at this moment they don't need to put anything into it, or even to fix it. It's okay as it is.

It is important to point out an underlying notion of health and illness here. The concepts of health and illness are a little bit like mind and body. We don't really know what we mean by health. Most of the research in Western medicine has been on illness; there is no funding for research on health. We might think that health is the absence of illness, but it's not that clear because there are obviously levels of health. The health of a twenty-year-old is not the same as the health of a seventy-year-old. Health can also include illness. For example, mothers may want their children to get measles to gain immunity to the disease. Illness can actually lead to greater health, so it's a dynamic balance.

This is a new view in the West. The old view was that illness is bad, and if we just destroy illness, then we'll have health. But it's much more complicated than that, especially because many of the illnesses we suffer from in the West are chronic illnesses related to lifestyle. In order to heal, you can't just go in and replace all the plumbing that breaks down. A lot of people would like to, because they get a lot of money for those operations. Bypass surgery, for example, is a very expensive operation, but it also bypasses the problem. The arteries are blocked for biological reasons; if you remove the blockage and replace it with a clean tube without changing the fundamental reasons for the illness, you haven't healed anything. However, there is new evidence in behavioral medicine that a combination of meditation, yoga, exercise, and a vegetarian diet can reverse even very severe heart disease. The coronary arteries that are blocked start to open, without drugs or surgery, and more blood flows to the heart. The mind's ability to change one's lifestyle is extremely powerful.

After teaching the body scan and introducing sitting meditation, we expand the field of the sitting meditation to focus on an object other than the body. Sound, or feeling states, or the flow of thoughts are good objects for meditation. If you watch a thought, it has a life of its own. As it dissolves you just continue observing, not following the chain of thoughts. In observing thought as the primary object in the meditation, we encourage people to do this for very short periods. It's very strenuous for beginners to be aware of thoughts as events in the field of consciousness, just arising in waves.

We end the sitting meditations with a technique called choiceless awareness, which is really a formless meditation with no object, just pure awareness. This is very difficult. We do not expect people to do this for long periods, but we include it just briefly to give a sense that it's possible to move from very specific objects to a much larger field. For instance, you can develop the flexibility to move from clearly and dispassionately seeing thoughts to being aware of sensations, and discerning that these are not the same thing.

We also do hatha yoga, which is a wonderful system for full-body strengthening and conditioning, and for developing flexibility and harmony in the body. Yoga, as you well know, means different things to different people. Very often it's used with no wisdom at all, out of greed or narcissism. We teach hatha yoga with mindfulness, so it's a form of Buddhist meditation without the Buddhism. Many people who come to our program have never used their bodies. They drive cars all the time and live a very sedentary lifestyle without much exercise. Physical therapists have a saying, "If you don't use it, you lose it." This applies not just to muscles, but also to the blood vessels, the joints, and so forth. Movement is very, very good for people. So we want to teach people to be mindful of their bodies not just in stillness but also in motion. This requires forms of meditation that involve moving with full awareness. Hatha yoga is very good for this.

ANXIETY: PHYSICAL AND MENTAL

I did a study in collaboration with Dan Goleman, who developed the Cognitive Somatic Anxiety questionnaire to measure anxiety. This is a way of determining whether people feel anxiety more in the mind or in the body. For instance, some people feel stress as butterflies in the stomach or a jittery feeling in the body, while others respond cognitively with anxious thoughts. We had noticed that some people liked the body scan but hated the sitting meditation. Other people loved the yoga but hated the body scan. Once people have learned sitting meditation, the body scan, and the yoga, we ask them how much they like each on a scale of one to a hundred. The sitting meditation is the most cognitive of these techniques, because you're just watching the mind without doing anything with the body. The body scan is more somatic; you're moving through the body mentally as you scan it. The yoga is the most somatic because you're actually moving the body. The people with high cognitive and low somatic anxiety like the yoga the most. They like the focus on the body, and it helps them because they are usually so much in their heads. On average, they like the body scan a little bit less and the sitting meditation less than that, although they still like them a lot. The people who feel anxiety more in the body than in the head like the sitting meditation best and the yoga least.

In this way, we can get a sense of why some people at least prefer one technique to another. One of the reasons we use different meditation techniques is to get as many people as possible to like one of them. Ideally, you want to teach people a method they will like, because if they don't like it, they won't do it as much. Their preference doesn't matter to us. We make them do all the techniques anyway, because there are some things they can learn from one that they won't learn from another. Sometimes you have to do things you don't like that may be good for you.

We also teach some informal mindfulness practices. These

are not techniques so much as ways of being. We want the development of moment-to-moment awareness to permeate all aspects of life, so we focus on tuning into the breathing throughout the whole day. Likewise, the very first thing we do to introduce people to meditation in the first class is not the body scan or breathing, but an eating meditation. This is a Theravada tradition I learned from my *vipassana* teachers. We pass out three raisins and eat them one at a time, five minutes per raisin, with full awareness: seeing, moving, tasting, taking onto the tongue, bringing it in, biting down, feeling the explosion of taste. You can probably taste it right now yourself, just in your imagination. Eating is one of the things that Westerners do more mindlessly than anything else. Many of our patients have weight problems. They eat because they're anxious or depressed, for emotional reasons—not because the body is hungry, but because the mind is hungry. This kind of eating out of greed never satisfies, and no wisdom develops around it. By bringing mindfulness into eating, we try to develop a whole new way of seeing.

We also teach standing meditation. When you're waiting for the bus, for example, why not just be mindful of standing: the feeling of the feet in contact with the ground, the body, the breath, and so forth. The next time you're standing in a long line in a store, instead of being impatient, just go into your standing meditation. The same goes for walking and other routine activities. We do washing-the-dishes meditation, taking-out-the-garbage meditation, cleaning-the-house meditation, taking-a-shower meditation. Right speech meditation includes mindfulness of actual talking: tone of voice, distance from the other person, listening, and so forth.

In the third week of the program, we have people tune in to pleasant events. Again, since we're such masters of mindlessness, often when we have pleasant feelings we don't even notice them, although we are very good at noticing the unpleasant feelings. One homework assignment is to notice a pleasant event every day for a week, and to really be there for it. If they forget to be there, they can remember it later, but ideally they should be fully mindful of it in the present moment, aware of sensations in the body, thoughts in the mind, feelings, and what the actions are that follow from this.

MINDFULNESS IN CHALLENGING SITUATIONS

The following week we get into stress and unpleasant events. We focus on perceiving stressors—the things in life that cause stress—with mindfulness of the body, thoughts, feelings, and actions. You just become aware of them; you don't have to do anything about them. Let's say someone hostile or angry causes you to have a strong reaction. You try to bring moment-to-moment awareness to the entire interchange without reacting. Of course, in the early stages you do react. However, as people develop more stability and calm in the formal meditation practice, they start to report that spontaneously they find themselves much calmer in situations that used to bother them a lot. Instead of reacting, they are developing more mindful responses. The continuity of awareness is protecting them from the stress reaction. This can be a very useful skill for people with severe coronary disease. We see many people in the clinic who have been told, "If you don't learn how to handle stress, the next time you have a heart attack, you're going to die." It's important for them to avoid a full-blown fight-or-flight reaction that increases their blood pressure.

Part of what we teach is to help people change their view of things. If we are constantly running around on automatic pilot, we have very little awareness of some of the things that are most important to us. For instance, many people in their fifties and sixties feel sadness because when their children were young, they really didn't pay attention to them from the heart. They were too busy with work, or they treated their children the way they had been treated, forgetting how painful it was to them. Our child-rearing practices may be one reason for our low self-esteem, although I don't want to oversimplify this.

To communicate that we want to challenge or expand the way the patients see things, we give them a puzzle as home-work in the first week. There are three parallel rows of three dots each, and the idea is to connect all nine dots with four straight lines without lifting the pen and without retracing. Many people get very upset and experience a lot of stress over it. Sometimes they struggle with it all week. When they can't solve it, they often get very judgmental and angry. They blame the problem, or they blame themselves and feel ashamed. That's not at all our motivation for doing this.

The mind has a way of seeing what it thinks is the problem, and often it's not the whole problem. It sees the nine dots as a square, and it doesn't see the context of the problem. The nervous system, the whole visual apparatus, and our habits of thinking make us very quick to focus in, and we don't stop to ask what the entire context of the problem is. Once you open up the field of attention or awareness, then new options and new solutions become possible. Even if you didn't get it, there's no need to blame yourself.

This is important for problem solving. If you have a very strong mentality, you persevere at a problem when you get stuck. But very often, the solution to a problem comes from penetrative awareness and looking at it freshly. This is part of scientific creativity. After you look at the problem for a while, you just let go of it and then a new picture appears with an expanded field.

A CASE HISTORY

I want to talk about the results of the clinic for one patient, a woman who was fifty-four years old when she came to us. She died some years ago of lupus, an autoimmune disease in which the immune system attacks parts of the body, but she was referred by her cardiologist because she had serious heart disease. She had a bypass operation on one artery, but two other major arteries in the heart were inoperable. She also had very high blood pressure and arthritis of the joints, and she was allergic to many drugs.

She often had to come into the hospital because of her lupus, which is a very difficult condition to treat. Sometimes her face and body would swell up beyond recognition because of the very strong steroids and other drugs she was taking. Often, the doctors could not tell her when she would get out of the hospital, which caused great turmoil and sadness in her life. She might come in before Thanksgiving and still be there at Christmas. Eventually, she was able to use meditation to reach a point of deep equanimity, being at peace with her disease.

Her blood pressure, which was very high at the time of her bypass surgery, dropped over the course of the stress-reduction program and then remained lower. We followed up for a number of years afterward, and it stayed down to the point where she was finally able to come off the medication and completely regulate her blood pressure using these techniques. When she started the program, she also had very disturbed sleep. Later, after eight or nine weeks, she started sleeping better.

This woman had an experience while she was doing the body scan as homework. About two weeks into the course, she had told me in class that she had no problem at all going through the body up to the neck area, but at that point she felt blocked and could not move on to the head. I told her not to worry, just go through the shoulders, or go around the neck outside the body. She tried this and was able to go around the block and up to the top of the head.

It was during that next body scan meditation that she heard the word "genitals" on the tape. She had been using the tape for two weeks before she ever heard the word. It's on the tape, and she had played it over and over, but she had selectively blocked it. Cognitive psychologists believe that we actually create our own reality by selectively filtering information from both the outside and the inside all the time. She did not hear this word until that day.

When she did hear it, it triggered a flashback of an experience that she had completely suppressed. She remembered that her father had regularly abused her sexually when she was between the ages of four and nine. She had repressed this. She was a fifty-four-year-old woman who had five children and who had been in therapy at that point for ten years, but she had not come close to this. For whatever reasons, the body scan triggered this memory. Following that was the clear memory of another scene. When she was nine years old, her father had died, and she was in the living room of their house with him at the time. He had a heart attack and fell on the floor. She was so frightened that she cowered in the corner. You can imagine her mixed feelings, because she loved her father but he was also her tormentor. Her mother came in after a while and blamed the girl for her father's death because she had not come to get her. She took a broom and beat the child violently around the head and neck.

This is the kind of suffering I believe many, many people are carrying around. Many of the people we see had experiences as children that were so deeply painful, the only way to deal with them was to shut them off. Now, forty years later, we're getting much more sophisticated about recognizing these problems and teaching children how to ask for help in these situations, but in those days you never talked about it.

When she had this flashback, she called me up, she wrote me a letter, and she came into the hospital, all on the same day. It was a very important experience for her. She increased her psychotherapy sessions as a result of this, and in the process joined a group for incest survivors. She continued her meditation practice, and later reached a point where she really valued the entire experience. For her, it was an unbelievable discovery, and then a liberation. When I first met her, her medical record was a stack of papers three feet high. She had heart disease, high blood pressure, arthritis, lupus, allergies, and all sorts of musculoskeletal problems. I believe very strongly, and a lot of evidence concurs, that when you repress this kind of pain as a child, it throws off the inner balance and harmony of the body—dysregulates the body on a profound level—and it comes out as disease.

This is the story of one person out of hundreds of our patients. They don't all have such a dramatic flashback experience, but by the time the eight weeks are over, the majority feel they have made contact with something deep inside themselves they never knew was there, and they feel very, very good about it. They often say it puts them in touch with feeling states they have not had since childhood, and a sense of belonging, or of their life being more their own.

When we started the program, we questioned whether ordinary Americans would be at all willing to practice meditation in any form, and we didn't know if throwing in yoga would make it seem even crazier. The answer is, after more than fifteen years, not only are mainstream Americans willing to practice this in a disciplined way at least for the eight weeks, but they actually love it.

MEDICAL EFFECTS OF
MINDFULNESS MEDITATION

I'd like to go very briefly now through some general results of the stress reduction program. We did a study over a two-year period of almost twelve hundred people who were referred to our clinic by their doctors. First, we wanted to know how many people actually get through the course and how many people drop out, because this is one measure of how good a clinic is. Of the 1,155 patients who were referred to us in two years, we had initial interviews with 75 percent. The remainder didn't want to come for one reason or another, or we couldn't get in touch with them. Of the people we interviewed, 90 percent enrolled in the program. Of those who enrolled, 92 percent actually started. Of those who started, 86 percent finished. These are very, very good results, especially because we work these people very hard. We say that it's stressful to take the stress reduction program, because it's a major lifestyle change to do nothing for forty-five minutes a day. We must be doing something they really appreciate, or they would not stay.

To put this in context, the usual rate of patients who keep a single doctor's appointment is 25 percent. People are notorious for not showing up for doctors' appointments, so it's asking a lot for them to stay in a program where they have to practice forty-five minutes a day, six days a week, plus spending the rest of their waking day in informal mindfulness practice. We ask a lot of people and we get a lot from them, and I think they enjoy this challenge.

If we take all people who were referred over a period of time with various pain problems, and we look at the number of different medical symptoms they report, there is a reduction of 25 percent in the number of symptoms over the eight weeks of the course. If we look at psychological symptoms, such as anger, anxiety, depression, and somatization, or imagining the body to be much worse than it is, we see a reduction of 32 percent in the number of symptoms over eight weeks. These people have had their pain problem for about eight years on the average, and have not previously been very successful at controlling their problem.

We also wanted to find out if they change on a more fundamental level. Almost anything can reduce symptoms for a short time. I could get up and do a dance, and their symptoms would go away for a while; or they might feel a little better if they just got together and talked. We wanted to know if anything more profound was happening, so we looked at measures of personality factors that supposedly increase resistance to stress. These are views that enable people to cope with stress, like the monks you mentioned whose inner view of the world helped them survive imprisonment and very hard conditions with few deep psychological scars. Someone else going through the same experience without those strong psychological factors might not survive at all, or might be too damaged to conduct daily life. Some of these measures were developed through studying concentration camp survivors from Germany. Compassion is one of the measures. Another is a sense of coherence, meaning that on some level you have a strong sense of understanding what's happening to you, however horrible it is. This is related to self-efficacy: you believe that you can somehow endure and find meaning in the experience. These are deep personality structures that supposedly do not change, certainly not in eight weeks. But we found that the average level on the sense-of-coherence scale for our patients increased by 7 percent during the program. This may not seem like much, but researchers in personality psychology say that a mean change of 7 percent is enormous. So not only are the symptoms decreasing, deeper psychological factors are actually changing.

A similar increase is found for the measure known as stress hardiness, which comprises three things: a sense of control, a commitment to the vividness of daily life experience, and the ability to deal with change as a challenge. For many people, change is a very big stress. Just when you feel comfortable, things change and you don't know where you are. If you learn to understand impermanence and flow more mindfully through change, then you can see it as a challenge and not necessarily as an obstacle. The results again show about a 6 percent change. This is preliminary evidence suggesting a major improvement in the deep structure of the mind. One would have to do much more sophisticated studies, some of which I will show, to determine whether these things are really important. But there is a suggestion that a major change is happening in these pain patients, not just at the level of their pain and psychological problems but also at the level of the deeper way in which they view the world. This comes back in some way to the puzzle of the nine dots. Something about their view of themselves in relationship to the world is changing. They feel more connected, more complete, and better able to go out and work with their pain without letting it undermine and damage their sense of vitality.

Oneness motive, which means a sense of belonging or connectedness, is another measure that shows similar improvement. We abbreviate it as OM, which I like. We measure oneness motive in a different way, so it's less likely to have the same kinds of bias as other measures. Instead of using a questionnaire, people write a story in response to a picture. Psychologists analyze the story for a particular kind of motivation that reflects oneness, or the deep feeling of unity. In a control group of people who were studied for eight weeks before they began the meditation training, measures for oneness motive did not change. There was a big increase in oneness motive when they went through the meditation training. Oneness motive, and other sophisticated psychological measures of motivation such as affiliative trust, have been linked with favorable immunological changes in other studies that we did with Dr. David McClelland at Harvard University.

GENERALIZATION OF EFFECTS FOR MINDFULNESS MEDITATION

Each time we do the program, we get the same results. Between the beginning and the end of the program, there is a sharp reduction in the number of both medical symptoms and psychological symptoms such as anxiety, anger, hostility, and somatization. In follow-up studies of patients who took the meditation training, the number of symptoms remains low over the four years of the study, so there is some evidence that the improvement is maintained over time. We question them a great deal about their meditation practice: whether they are still meditating, how much, how long, what techniques they use, whether they do the informal practices such as mindfulness in daily life, and so forth. Ninety-three percent say that four years later, they are still doing something that they learned in the program. Forty-five percent are continuing to practice the formal meditation daily for at least fifteen minutes at a time, at least three times a week. Four years have passed with no reinforcement.

There is a big difference between men and women in response to the training when they come for chronic pain problems. More women respond positively than men, and this may have to do with work-related issues. The women may have more motivation for getting better than the men. However, this is not true for patients who have problems other than pain, such as stress-related heart disease or cancer. It seems to be peculiar to pain that women do better than men. The results show that for pain, the frequency and the severity of the pain, the number of medical symptoms, and the psychological distress all decrease. The personality measures of stress hardiness and sense of coherence both improve.

If we look at diagnoses for individual diseases, we see the same kind of changes resulting from the meditation training: a reduction of 40 to 45 percent in medical symptoms, a similar if not greater reduction in psychological distress, and increases of 4 to 8 percent in the personality measures that buffer against stress. Heart disease, high blood pressure, and digestive problems show the same general pattern, so the pattern is independent of the diagnosis. Over 80 percent of the people report a certain level of reduction in physical and psychological symptoms. Not every single person responds favorably to the meditation practice. The 15 or 20 percent who do not just don't connect up with the meditation in a good way; they don't understand why this is happening and why we're not fixing them.

It's very hard to have an adequate control group when you run a clinic, but sometimes you make comparisons with patients from other clinics who are referred in a similar process. In this way, we have done a number of controlled studies, and found that other clinics using medical interventions do not get such good results with similar patients who have the same kinds of pain problems. Something about mobilizing the mind in addition to the medical treatments is better than the medical treatments alone.

MINDFULNESS AND THE TREATMENT OF SPECIFIC DISORDERS

We did one particular study in collaboration with the department of psychiatry. Some people suffer from spontaneous panic attacks that are not caused by anything in the external environment. It is a well-known clinical syndrome: they lose control completely and are very frightened; their heart rate and blood pressure go way up; they may think they're having a heart attack; they may have a hard time breathing. We wanted to see how well people with panic disorder do in this meditation training. (Most of our patients are not referred from psychiatry, but from general medicine and various medical specialties.) We wanted to let another group of people test our patients to avoid bias. So our psychiatrist colleagues tested these people. The anxiety ratings for these patients started at a high level and then began to go down when the program started. There was a little blip at around six weeks, when we had our all-day session and people were very frightened about being in a room for eight hours without talking, and then it decreased again. We followed them for three months after the program ended, and it tended to stay down. These results were achieved without any drugs. They are as good as, if not better than, results shown with people who are being given drugs for genuine panic disorder. Anxiety and panic often go hand in hand with depression, and we see the exact same pattern for depression.

Over the years, many doctors have become very interested in meditation, and we have worked with different specialists, including pulmonary doctors. It's very nice to have the pulmonary doctors collaborating with the meditation clinic, looking at breathing in two different ways. Chronic obstructive pulmonary disease, or COPD, is a common problem in the United States, caused almost entirely by smoking, or in some cases by breathing toxic chemicals in the workplace. People lose elasticity in the lungs and can't breathe very well. The shortness of breath can in turn cause agitation and panic. We train people in the pulmonary rehabilitation program in mindfulness. We teach them to become more friendly with their breathing through daily meditation practice, and they begin to realize they do not have to panic when they have an episode of shortness of breath. In consequence, their experiences of shortness of breath decrease in frequency and severity, and their confidence in their ability to handle it increases, which leads to further improvement. Meditation training and mindfulness have become the cornerstone of this entire pulmonary rehabilitation clinic.

We're also working in a dermatology clinic. There is a common skin disease called psoriasis. It's somewhat genetic, but not well understood, and it gets worse with stress. The skin cells grow too fast and the skin becomes flaky in certain places, or it can cover the whole body. The treatment involves standing with your eyes covered in a box that looks like a telephone booth lined with ultraviolet light bulbs. The ultraviolet light prevents the cells from dividing and slows their growth. We thought, if they were just standing there for a period of time, why not teach them standing meditation? We thought they might heal more quickly if we included the mind as a factor. The speed of healing is important because exposure to the ultraviolet light increases the risk of skin cancer. We had them listen to a tape through headphones as they stood under the light with no clothes on, visualizing the light hitting the skin and the cells slowing down their growth.

We compared two groups, those who had only the regular medical light treatment, and those who did meditation in addition to the light treatment. The survival curve shows that of those who received only the light treatment, none healed completely. Most take forty weeks for the symptoms to clear halfway. The statistics show very powerfully even for this small study that the meditators clear much faster than the nonmeditators.

A more powerful treatment uses a drug taken orally in combination with the ultraviolet light. In another study, again of a small group, all the meditators cleared by thirty weeks, more quickly than the nonmeditators. I want to emphasize that this does not prove anything: it's a suggestion that the mind might play a role in this healing process. We are now collaborating with other centers that have many more psoriasis patients, introducing meditation in their dermatology clinics. It's too early to say for sure, but if this turns out to be true, we could do some very interesting studies. We could use light without ultraviolet wavelengths to study the effect of the mind alone. We could also study the role of the immune system in psoriasis, and the mind's effects on epidermal growth factor and other gene-control systems in the skin. It's a very nice experimental system with a clear meditation input.

People who come through our meditation clinic tend to continue to practice for a long time afterward. Sometimes they continue to practice even when they don't improve. We followed up on some pain patients who had experienced no reduction of pain at all, and yet many of these people continued to meditate three years later. When we ask them why, they say they are learning other things through the meditation practice that help them live with the pain in some way. There too, we're killing two birds with one stone. If the pain decreases, it's great; but it's counterproductive to strive for the pain to decrease. When people come into the program, we tell them to leave their expectations at the door and just keep focused on moment-to-moment awareness and looking deeply into themselves. Although we see big improvements, very often the most important thing people get out of the program was not what they came looking for. They find something deeper.

When we ask what they found in the meditation training program, they mention two things. One I think is very funny: they say "the breathing." I ask, "What do you mean? You were breathing for many years before you began meditation." What they mean is they have a new-found awareness of the special quality of breath that relates to a greater sensitivity and awareness of their whole body. Along with the breath comes a sense of greater appreciation for the miracle of having a body, even if the body has a disability. Each breath, each moment, is a miracle, and when you begin to experience that directly, it vitalizes the quality of your life because you stop missing or running through so many of your moments. The other thing they say is, "I learned that I am not my thoughts, and by extension I learned that I am not my pain or my suffering."

Mindfulness and Medical Training

I'd like now to move to the question of medical education, not just of medical students, but also of doctors. Doctors have a lot of stress, and they make sure the medical students also have a lot of stress: "We had to learn medicine a certain way, so you have to learn it the same way." Medical education is not as good as it could be in developing people who are strong in compassion, empathy, humility, and equanimity. Doctors have to work with people who have the worst possible suffering, and yet they don't receive training in this. We have started to train medical students and interested physicians in mindfulness as a way of helping them improve the communication and interaction between doctor and patient.

We are teaching these listening skills to the medical students now because the doctor/patient relationship is extremely important for healing. Very often the doctor can do more with his or her being than with drugs, so physicians really need to learn the medical art of close listening, compassion, and awareness. When they graduate from medical school, they usually hear a speech about compassion, humility, and equanimity, but no one ever teaches them how to develop these qualities. In the Tibetan tradition, if you want to develop compassion or equanimity, you work at it for thirty or forty years. In the West, we talk about these beautiful ideals at graduation ceremonies, but no one ever bothers to tell you how to develop them.

When the students arrive, I am the first person they meet in their first two days at medical school. I tell them about meditation and the role of the mind in health and illness, and try to establish from the very beginning a foundation in an alternative view—a larger view that suggests they should protect themselves while they are in medical school so that in the process of becoming a doctor, they don't forget who they are and why they wanted to become a doctor in the first place. This can be a very serious problem. If you suspend your own life while you're working hard to get something you want, by the time you get it, you may not know why you wanted it. Doctors in the United States have very high rates of suicide and alcohol and drug abuse because they suffer from a lot of stress for which they don't have adequate training.

So we now train medical students in a stress-reduction program that lasts eight weeks, just like that for the patients. It's not as intensive, only fifteen minutes of meditation daily for homework, because they don't have time for forty-five minutes. When the eight weeks are over, they don't want to stop, so we continue for eight months, but this is optional. They get no credit or exams, and homework and class attendance are not compulsory. The course is based on love, on caring for this vital principle of life and awareness itself. It's very popular because of that. We also have an elective in which they can observe the clinic itself and watch the patients. We also train doctors, residents, and interns, as well as the medical students. We're trying to introduce meditation and the whole notion of the connection of mind and body into medical education.

The theoretical physicist David Bohm points out in his book, *Wholeness and the Implicate Order,* that the words *meditation* and *medicine* share the same Indo-European root. In Latin, *mederi* means to cure, but the root meaning is actually to measure. You might wonder what medicine or meditation have to do with measure. Nothing, if we think of measure as an external standard like a ruler. But the root refers to a more Platonic notion of right inward measure, the properties that make something what it is. The body's right inward measure is health, when everything is in balance. So medicine is the restoring of right inward measure when there is a lack of balance; and meditation is the direct perception of right inward measure. I find it useful to challenge the medical students to think about these things on a deeper level, and to understand the notions of wholeness and unity that may help them avoid being too reductionist about the disease process.

Notes

1. *Anatman* literally means not-self, egolessness. In Buddhism, the realization of egolessness is fundamental to enlightenment.

2. The three marks of existence are basic postulates of Buddhism: impermanance (*anitya*), suffering *(dukha)*, and egolessness (*anattama*).

7

Behavioral Medicine

DANIEL BROWN

OVER THE PAST thirty years, discoveries in biology and psychology have led to a synthesis of ideas about using the ability of the mind to produce healing changes in the body as the scientific evidence has grown that emotional states influence physical health for better or worse. One prominent version of this integration is behavioral medicine, the application of techniques such as biofeedback, relaxation training, and hypnosis to the treatment of medical and psychosomatic disorders.

These methods are used to treat a wide range of medical problems, from headaches and chronic pain to hypertension, asthma, and even adverse reactions to other medical treatments like chemotherapy. Behavioral medicine is also used to treat unhealthy habits and addictions, such as overeating, substance abuse, and smoking, as well as to enhance personal well-being by helping people relax and focus their minds. Daniel Brown reviews the methods of behavioral medicine, with examples from his own clinical practice.

D A N I E L   B R O W N :   Behavioral medicine has developed a number of treatment approaches, including self-monitoring, self-regulation, calming or relaxation therapy, heightening internal perception, and cognitive therapy, which challenges self-defeating thoughts. All these approaches are based on learning theory, which involves teaching the body to develop healthy habits and to reverse the negative learning of bad habits. As a result, the body achieves a new kind of balance, or self-regulation.

Self-monitoring is one of the approaches that we typically use. We ask people to keep daily records or diaries of their symptoms. For example, if a person has chronic pain, we ask them to record their experience of pain hourly in a diary, and rate the pain on a scale from zero for no pain to five for excruciating pain. They would also write down for each hour what they were doing, their situation, and their thoughts and feelings at the time. They would keep this diary for two weeks.

By having people monitor themselves, we are training them to observe themselves skillfully. This increases their awareness of the symptoms and also the context. If they keep track of the changing intensity of the pain, after a while they begin to see relationships between the situation and the increase or decrease in pain. Then, we have them identify high-risk times. For example, if the pain is always very intense at eight o'clock each morning, that would be considered a high-risk time. If it's always intense on weekends but not during the week, then we have them identify high-risk situations. Maybe the pain is worse when they're in some sort of conflict at work.

Stimulus control, which is based on learning theory, is another method we use. When people have a bad habit, after a while that habit becomes associated with neutral events that will trigger it through learning. For example, some people may eat excessively as a bad habit. Every time they see food around the house, or see an advertisement for food, they automatically start eating. After a while, the environment shapes the habit.

Insomnia is another example. There may be a short-term

cause: a person is worried about an exam, or the weather has warmed, so he or she opens the windows and hear the sounds outside. Typically, the cause goes away when the stressful situation ends, usually after a few days or a week. But people worry about going to sleep, so they start reading or watching television in bed, or they bring food into the bedroom. What makes people go to sleep is shutting off information from the world and letting the body become inactive. When you lie down and close your eyes, the lack of movement and sudden shift from taking in stimulation from the outside activate a mechanism for the brain to go to sleep. If you keep the central nervous system active by reading or watching television, you can't sleep. So the very behavior that a person used to handle the problem of not sleeping now causes the problem. If we give people very simple instructions to take the television out of the bedroom, to go into the bedroom only when it's time to sleep or when they're tired, we find that 70 percent of people with sleep problems show improvement within five sessions. The implication is that a lot of insomnia is caused by this kind of environmental shaping and learning. Stimulus control treatment takes into account how the environment or the context maintains the problem.

Another technique is called behavioral self-regulation. Suppose people have a problem like smoking. We begin the treatment by having them self-monitor the smoking behavior. They write down every time they have a cigarette, rating how much they needed the cigarette on scale of one to five. Again, they keep this diary for two weeks. Then we have them work out a schedule to cut out the least-needed cigarettes, until they achieve that goal. Then we set a new goal, cutting all the cigarettes rated the next stage higher. Eventually the only cigarettes they're smoking are those most needed, and then we work out a way of handling those too. In this kind of self-regulation, we work with a schedule and establish criteria, setting goals. People will pursue their own goals if you set them low enough, because they take great pride in mastering a goal and then going onto the next goal. Through that they learn to change their behavior.

Relaxation Therapy and Skillful Internal Perception

Relaxation therapy or calming is another method we use. This can be done by systematically tensing and relaxing each of the muscle groups in the body, a technique called progressive muscle relaxation. It can also be done through hypnosis and through meditation of various kinds. We also use different kinds of breathing exercises and biofeedback.

As part of the method called skillful internal perception, we ask ordinary people in the West, not yogis or meditators, to observe changes in the internal bodily state. We find that most people are very inaccurate in their observations. Surprisingly, most people can give a fairly accurate estimate of general physiological changes, like blood pressure and blood sugar levels, but most are very poor at picking up specific changes. If we ask the ordinary person to tell us what muscles are involved in a headache, usually they get it wrong. If you ask someone with irritable bowel syndrome to tell when they have too much activity of the muscles that make up the intestine, they can't say with any accuracy.

People with certain problems are especially poor in the ability to discriminate. For example, most people who have weight problems often confuse emotions with hunger. They tend to eat when they feel anxiety or sadness, because they misperceive the emotion as hunger. About 80 percent of people who have asthma cannot tell how much the muscles of their lungs are contracted. To gain control over these physiological processes, we teach people how to be aware of them.

The last major treatment is cognitive therapy. We teach people to become aware of the thoughts that go through the mind, to write them down and identify the habitual negative thoughts, and then to develop an antidote. The antidote takes the form of affirmations or positive thoughts that they make an effort to repeat during the day, almost like a mantra, to break up the habitual negative pattern. People can actually think themselves into an asthma attack or a headache, so we have to break up that pattern.

HEADACHES: A DETAILED LOOK AT TREATMENT WITH BEHAVIORAL MEDICINE

About 60 percent of the people who come to our outpatient department come in with headaches; it's our most frequent referral. There are three major kinds of headaches that we understand. The first has a strong biological basis to it, such as the headache that accompanies a tumor or an illness like the flu or other infection, or the headache that comes with a hangover. These are all examples of headaches caused by the release of chemicals in the body or by tissue changes. We can't treat these headaches with behavioral medicine, but they constitute perhaps only 5 percent of all the cases that come to the clinics. The other two types are muscle tension headaches and vascular headaches. Muscle tension headaches, caused primarily by the contraction of muscles within the head, neck, and scalp, are the most common, accounting for about 85 percent of all headaches. Vascular headaches are caused by changes in the blood flow. Most people who come to our clinic have a mixture of muscle tension and vascular headaches, not just one or the other.

Treatment needs to involve both the factors that caused the headache and those that maintain it. Any of the types of stress mentioned earlier can cause headaches by producing changes in the muscle tension level and blood flow. People who have chronic headaches have certain bands of muscles in the head, neck, and scalp that remain contracted; the high levels of muscle tension are there all the time, even when they're free of headaches. If they're under stress, then a little bit more change causes perception of the pain. That muscle tissue is different from healthy muscle tissue. It's much harder to the touch because it's filled with fluid from a build-up of certain saccharides in the tissue.

There are also changes in the blood flow patterns of the vasomotor system. When a person is vulnerable to a vascular headache, like a migraine headache, there is a characteristic pattern of changes in the size of the blood vessels that goes along with the headache. First the blood vessels in the skin constrict, typically in response to some sort of stress. The constriction of the blood vessels in the skin is a prodrome, an early warning phase. For some people this constriction also extends to the cranial arteries and interferes with blood flow to the brain, causing changes in visual perception or even nausea. These early symptoms indicate a classic migraine headache. About twenty minutes to half an hour later, the cranial arteries expand. That's the point at which the person starts to report the headache.

When the cranial arteries expand, a series of biochemical changes occurs. The platelets, which are cells floating in the bloodstream, stick together and then release catecholamines into the bloodstream and the tissue. These chemicals are part of the body's stress-response cycle. They in turn release other chemicals that lower the pain threshold, so the person becomes more sensitive to the perception of pain. The tissue becomes inflamed; this is a sterile inflammatory response similar to the inflammation caused by bacterial infection. That's why people who have vascular headaches have very intense pain that can last for hours and sometimes even several days. The release of these biochemicals makes the pain more intense and inflames the tissue.

Once the headache forms, there are a number of factors that can make it continue over time. For example, worrying about the headache itself can cause dysregulation of the autonomic nervous system, which causes the muscle and blood flow changes that set up the whole pattern. Headaches can be conditioned, so the whole pathway can happen without the stress. People who keep diaries in the first year that they have headaches can usually identify an event that causes the headache about 70 percent of the time. If those same people keep diaries five years later, they can only identify events that caused 30 percent of their headaches. Ten years later, they can identify causes for less than 10 percent. The whole physiological response pattern becomes conditioned, and all the changes occur with very little provocation from an external event. People who have had headaches for five or ten years say they don't know what causes them any more, they just happen, and in fact they do. That's why we have to appreciate the role of learning in understanding these headaches.

One of the first things we do with a headache patient is to have him or her keep a daily diary. We find that for any given patient with a headache, there are usually from four to six factors, some more important than others. After several weeks of monitoring, we can identify the risk pattern for that individual. Then we recommend changes in the factors associated with the headache.

They keep a headache diary on a series of cards with a picture of a head. They can color in or use numbers to indicate the area where they have a headache. It shows the hours of the day, and has a rating of headache intensity from no headache to a very severe headache. Each hour of the day they have to give a rating of how intense the headache is. The diary of one of my patients showed that when she woke up in the morning she had a very excruciating headache. It went down somewhat during the day, and then at night it came back.

If a person keeps a daily diary like this for several weeks, you can usually identify a pattern specific to that person, but it's not the same for everybody. So for that one patient, for example, there are certain high-risk times, morning and night. Then we have to ask, why is the pain worse in the morning and the evening and not during the day?

DALAI LAMA: In this case, is the patient working?

DANIEL BROWN: The patient is working. This particular patient is a mother, a single parent with three children who has to work and take care of these kids.

DALAI LAMA: So during the day her mind probably just gets distracted as she just thinks about other things? Would that account for a decrease in the headache?

DANIEL BROWN: We looked at this for several weeks: every time she has the pain, she's getting her children dressed and off to school, or fixing them breakfast or dinner. Almost every day you see the same pattern, so we've identified a high-risk situation. The pain is the worst whenever she's worried about getting her kids settled.

DALAI LAMA: How is she spending her time right there in the midpoint of the day when the headache is the least?

DANIEL BROWN: She's working.

DALAI LAMA: And not thinking about her children?

DANIEL BROWN: That's right. We wondered just as Your Holiness is wondering about it: what is the pattern?

Examples of typical physical causes of headaches are certain foods, including foods high in nitrites, and a variety of environmental factors, such as cigarette smoke or exhaust fumes from cars. Caffeine causes constriction of the blood vessels, and alcohol causes expansion of the blood vessels. If people use a lot of caffeine or alcohol, or both in combination, which is common, the blood vessels are constantly changing size, so they get less stable over time. In this case the person's behavior makes the headache worse. Hunger and fasting lower blood sugar levels, which can trigger headaches in some individuals. Hormonal changes around menstruation cause headaches for some women. Exercise can be a factor, also sometimes oversleep. When people lie awake in bed in the morning, their breathing gets very shallow, which reduces the amount of oxygenated blood going to the brain. This can trigger the blood flow changes because the blood vessels in the brain open more to adjust for this.

Some individuals are sensitive to changes in the cardiovascular system that are caused by repressing their anger. This is a factor only for about 20 percent of all people with vascular headaches. Headaches that have to do with emotions are much less common than we used to think. Medication abuse is another possibility. Ergot, derived from a common bread mold, is a medication that causes the blood vessels to constrict, so it is used to stop headaches caused by expansion of the cranial arteries. But people get worried about the headache coming on and take the medication unnecessarily, which makes the blood vessels less stable, so the very treatment then becomes the cause of the illness.

The next phase of the treatment is to identify the pattern of muscles where the spasm is, and for this we use an electromyograph. A muscle that is active or spasmed gives off much more electrical activity than one that is relaxed. We use a scanner, simply touching the electrode to the head and scalp, to get a reading of the muscle activity involved in a particular headache pattern for a given individual. We need an objective way of finding out exactly the muscles involved, because people often perceive referred pain at a point different from where the muscle tension is.

After we identify the pattern, then we use biofeedback. We put the electrodes on a particular muscle, and when its activity is above a certain level, the machine makes a blipping noise. When the spontaneous activity of the muscle drops below that level, the noise stops. We ask the person to make the machine be quiet, which is another way of saying to decrease the muscle activity. After the individual learns to do this, we repeat the process, setting the machine to give feedback at progressively lower levels of muscle activity. It usually takes five to ten sessions to learn to reduce a muscle's activity to normal, and we develop an individualized program to address each muscle that's high for an individual.

Treatment of Chronic Pain

One man came to our laboratory with chronic pain that was caused by an injury but had lasted for four or five years and prevented him from working. The reading we took of this muscle was five microvolts. When we asked him to make the

machine be quiet, it jumped up to almost ten. This person
didn't have any idea how to relax. He was trying very hard,
which made him less relaxed, and it got much worse. We
explained that you can't try to relax, that relaxation means
calming both the body and the mind, and it's something that
you have to let happen rather than make happen.

With some instruction, he began to become calm, and in
the same session he was able to drop the muscle level down
to three microvolts, learning voluntary control. In the next
biofeedback session, he was able to drop it down to about
two microvolts, and it continued dropping as he learned. At
first, the muscle activity was still high when he came in and
dropped during the session, but then gradually the learning
became generalized. By the seventh or eighth session, the
muscle activity remained low during the week. We also had
him keep a daily record of the pain, rating it from zero to
five, and then we averaged the ratings for each week. The
average for the first week was about four, which means very
intense pain. It decreased steadily so that by the eighth week
his pain estimate was generally very mild. There were times
during the week where it was still very high or low, but on
the average it was much less. As he taught the muscles to
relax, the pain perception also dropped.

When he felt confident enough to go back to work, the
muscle activity level and the pain both increased sharply, because the work was stressful for him. But he was able to generalize what he had learned and apply it to the new situation.
Two sessions later, he had taught the muscle to remain relaxed even in a high-stress situation, and the pain readings
went down again. At follow-up sessions after three months
and six months, there was no high muscle activity. The pain
was relatively mild and eventually disappeared.

So far I've talked about teaching the patient to gain control
over muscle activity, but that's only half the problem. We
also have to teach control over the blood flow patterns of the
vasomotor response. We use thermometers on your fingers
for this, because skin temperature is a function of the size of
the blood vessels. When the blood vessels are open, the in-

creased flow of warm blood raises the skin temperature. When the blood vessels are constricted, the temperature drops. The temperature is also related to stress, which causes the blood vessels to constrict. When a person is relaxed, the blood vessels open and the temperature goes up, so the temperature reading provides feedback. We ask people to see if they can make their hands get warm. They visualize warming their hands over an imaginary flame or a hot stove, or they imagine being out in the warm sunshine. After three to five minutes, they open their eyes to see if they've changed the temperature.

VISCERAL LEARNING: THE IMPORTANCE OF PRACTICE

In visceral learning, teaching the body a new physiological habit, the magnitude of the change is not as important as the consistency of practice. For the body to learn a new habit, doing a little bit each day is better than making a big change and then not doing anything for a few days. So we have people take the thermometers home and practice six times a day for three to five minutes. By producing a change of only two degrees, they become skilled at gaining voluntary control over the blood flow pattern, using the mind to control the body. Once they get skilled at doing this with the thermometers on the fingers of both hands, we then tape them to the hand. Then we move them to the wrist, and eventually they can change the temperature of the entire lower arm by one or two degrees. Once they can do that at will, we tape the thermometers on the toes, which are much harder to do, and then the feet. Gradually they learn to change the temperature of larger and larger surface areas of the body. The more skillful they become, the greater the likelihood for improvement of their headaches, because they're gaining control over the whole blood flow pattern. Since headache is caused by a local dysregulation of the blood flow, this puts things back into balance. On the average it takes about twenty weeks. Some people are much quicker and some are slower, but most people can learn this.

The next thing we teach people is diaphragmatic breathing exercises. They learn to breathe in and out slowly with the hands on the abdomen, using the expansion of the hands as feedback. When they do this regular breathing for about twenty minutes a day, it causes a rapid uptake of catecholamines. These are chemicals involved in the stress response cycle, so that the breathing actually helps prevent the build up of the very things that inflamed the tissue. While they're doing the breathing exercise, they focus on the movement of the diaphragm. If they do the breathing exercises while they actually have the headache, it makes it worse. Also, if they are shallow breathers, that can sometimes make it worse, so they have to be carefully instructed in the breathing exercises. If they do them correctly, over time it works preventatively so that the headaches become less frequent and less intense.

DISCOVERING THE SEQUENCE OF SYMPTOMS

The first part of the treatment is getting rid of bad physiological habits and teaching the body healthier responses, using the techniques of muscle relaxation, blood flow change, and breathing exercises. The next part of the treatment is to work with the acute headache while the symptoms are actually present. We try to identify the behavioral chain leading up to the headache. We ask the person to identify the earliest symptom before he or she actually feels the intense pain. Over time, people learn to identify earlier and earlier symptoms. For example, they might first feel a little funny; then ten minutes later, they notice some nausea and visual changes. Five or ten minutes after that, they realize a headache is coming on. There is a point of recognition, and then the negative thoughts begin: "Oh no, this is going to be the worst headache ever. Here we go again. There's nothing I'm going to be able to do about it." The negative thoughts make it much worse, and at this point they feel a lot of pain.

After we construct the behavioral chain of events, we have them work out healthy strategies to cope with each step. When they start feeling a little funny, they remind themselves to practice relaxation; calming themselves may prevent the headache from happening. If they notice changes in the visual field and also nausea, that's a good time to practice with the thermometers to voluntarily change the blood flow before the headache builds up. If they notice the negative thoughts coming, they can cut them off by reminding themselves of positive, confident things.

COPING STRATEGIES TO COUNTERACT THE SEQUENCE OF SYMPTOMS

Finally, they practice pain coping strategies. We teach people ways of attending that alter the actual perception of pain. We find that people are very different in their abilities to alter pain perception. There are essentially four different approaches, and what works for one person may not work for another. Some people can use avoidance: distracting themselves, fantasizing, thinking about something other than the pain, or focusing on outside events. Some people can alleviate the pain by imagining their hand getting numb, and then transferring the numbness to the location of the pain, like a visualization on lack of sensation. A third approach is to directly alter the perception of the pain, focusing on the pain and imagining it as a tingling sensation or warmth rather than pain. A fourth approach is mindfulness: to simply place the awareness fully on the pain until it shifts. We teach people whatever method works best for them, using a neutral pain that isn't an area of conflict for them, rather than the headache. We create the pain by simply pinching, and then assess different pain-coping strategies. Most people find one or two of these strategies will work for them, and then we apply them to alter the pain as they're actually having it.

An example of the results can be seen with the mother of three children who had the headaches in the morning and evening. She engaged in a daily practice of calming the body in general, doing breathing exercises, and working specifically with the muscles and blood flow in the head. But her pattern of headaches didn't change very much until about twenty weeks later—to the point where she didn't have any more headaches, after thirteen years of daily headaches. We followed up, and she did not have a headache for six years, until she got pregnant. The headaches came back then, but went away when she practiced, and she has not had a headache since.

DALAI LAMA: Wonderful. It worked.

DANIEL BROWN: So, this is a strong example of the learning, but it takes time to teach the body better habits.

REDUCING HYPERTENSION WITH BEHAVIORAL MEDICINE

We also use this same approach for treating hypertension, or high blood pressure. We start first by having people keep a diary of their blood pressure, which they measure three times a day, as a baseline. The steps in the treatment are general calming, followed by warming exercises, which are the most important part of the treatment: the hands, up the entire arm, and then the feet, for about twenty weeks. Patients use simple thermometers to measure the warming. We also do the breathing exercises. The treatment is similar to that for headaches because hypertension also has a lot to do with blood flow patterns.

One person came in with a systolic blood pressure of 180, which is high, and diastolic blood pressure of 100, also quite high. We wanted to get his diastolic pressure down from about 100 to about 80. When he started keeping a baseline for six weeks, there was a small drop in blood pressure simply as a result of observing it; the mindfulness already caused some change. At the end of the twentieth week of training, his diastolic blood pressure dropped from 100 to 82, and the systolic pressure also went down to about 150. Now 150 may seem high, but this is a 70-year-old.

Many of these patients are on medications already. During the treatment, we do not ask them to change their medications at first. For many patients, the effects of the drugs and the behavioral training eventually combine, dropping the blood pressure too quickly. They start getting symptoms of postural hypotension, getting dizzy when they sit up too quickly. At that point, we cut back the drugs and let them use the mind instead. Whenever the diastolic blood pressure drops below an average of eighty for two weeks, we cut the medications by 20 percent. If the pressure stays down, two weeks later we'll cut the medications by another 20 percent. If it goes back up, we'll adjust the medications again. About one-third of the patients can drop below the goal of eighty in a stable way with no medications. Another third can achieve this with a reduction of medication, and for another third this treatment doesn't work.

I chose the next example of a hypertensive patient for the benefit of our wonderful translators this week. This particular patient is an interpreter who works in the court system. This is a very stressful situation. He has to translate very accurately because his words are recorded into the legal record, and he always worries about getting it just right. During the self-monitoring, we identified that translating in court was the most important trigger that made his blood pressure rise. We taught him to practice, and the diastolic and systolic pressure dropped as a result. When he reached the goal of eighty, we then asked him to take the thermometers into the courtroom and practice during the free time. From then on he recorded his blood pressure only in this high-stress situation. Gradually he became skillful at lowering his blood pressure even in this most stressful situation. He's been able to generalize the learning to a new situation, applying the new habit not only in a calm state but also in a high-stress situation.

For the person who practices very inconsistently, often skipping a couple of days, the results are choppy. You can see a large difference if people practice regularly. The consistency of the change is more important than the magnitude. For the body to learn a new habit, doing a little bit each day is better than making a big change and then not doing anything for a few days.

THE TREATMENT OF ASTHMA

Asthma is a condition in which the smooth muscle tissue lining the air passages contracts in a spasm. The air is trapped inside the bronchial passages, so the person has difficulty breathing out. Asthma may be chronic or acute. In the chronic condition, some of the smaller branches of the airway passages contract. It varies over time, sometimes more, sometimes less, but a person who is vulnerable to asthma will have some degree of contraction much of the time.

An acute asthma attack is more than contraction of the small air passages. The main large air passage contracts and causes such an obstruction of the airflow that the person can't breathe, and it becomes a crisis. When we treat asthma behaviorally, we consider both the chronic small air spasm as well as the acute condition. We begin, again, with self-monitoring, teaching people to be aware when their air passages are more contracted and when they're less contracted. Most people perceive this poorly, so we use a device called a peak flow meter, which measures how much air you can force out with effort in a short amount of time. The peak flow meter is accurate but not very expensive, so people can take them home and keep a diary to monitor themselves. Again, for the first two or three weeks, we have them record a baseline. Many asthmatics show improvement already during this time. Because they start to recognize their own patterns, they don't worry so much in anticipation of an asthma attack. As they learn to accurately perceive the symptoms, the awareness training itself already has a beneficial effect.

That's the first step. Then we teach them relaxation and peak flow biofeedback. They use the peak flow meter while they do special breathing exercises, visualizing forcing the air out gently. If they try too hard the spasm increases, but if they're in a very relaxed state, they may be able to find just the right amount of effort so the bronchial spasm decreases and the reading goes up. They can teach themselves a certain breathing technique, which is often very individualized. They're teaching themselves voluntary control over the smooth muscle response. This doesn't work for asthma related to allergy and inflammation, but it is very effective for asthma related to stress symptoms.

PART FOUR

Emotion and Culture

EAST AND WEST

8

The Virtues in Christian and Buddhist Traditions

LEE YEARLEY

LEE YEARLEY compares characteristics of virtues and vices within the Christian and Confucian traditions, some of which are also part of the Buddhist tradition. He focuses on one particular schema of virtue and vice, that of Thomas Aquinas, a thirteenth-century Christian cleric. Dr. Yearley indicates that Aquinas's list of virtues and vices often resembles similar lists conceived by Buddhist and Confucian thinkers. Following this presentation, the Dalai Lama discusses the Buddhist conception of virtue, which evolves into a dialogue in which the motivation of action is considered, along with the action itself. Moral dilemmas are discussed, such as when violence is justified and when an action is nonvirtuous.

There are several general characteristics of virtues within the Christian and Confucian traditions, characteristics that are also part of the Buddhist tradition. Most traditions think virtues are examples of human excellence, of human flourishing. They are permanent additions to the self, key parts of people's character, aspects of what makes people who they are. Moreover, virtues are manifested not only in what one does but also in what one feels and desires; emotions are a very important aspect of them.

Virtues are also *corrective*. That is, virtues correct some difficulty thought to be natural to human beings, some temptation that needs to be resisted or some motivation that needs to be made good. Courage, for example, corrects the inclination to be stopped by fear from doing what should be done; in a similar fashion, compassion corrects the tendency to be selfish.

Another characteristic of virtues is that they are *expressive*. That is, they express a person's conception of what a good life is. A virtuous person, for example, tries to stop the vicious attacker about to hurt an innocent child just because the person believes the courage and compassion displayed in that act expresses what a good human life is. This feature of virtues means that virtuous activity and physical health may sometimes conflict. For example, expressing compassion and courage in the situation just described can bring physical harm, or even death.

Given these general characteristics, let us turn now to the virtues and vices Thomas Aquinas lists. I will start with the vices; they share all the characteristics of virtues except that they are aimed toward the bad rather than the good. That is, they reinforce rather than correct bad inclinations and express a flawed conception of the good life. Aquinas thinks seven vices or sins are especially important because they both are particularly dangerous and produce other sins. (They are often called the seven deadly sins.)

Lust is being guided by one's sexual desires in situations in which other considerations should be more prominent, such as paying attention to what ethics demands of you. Gluttony is the continuing desire to consume food or drink to such excess that you cease to care about other more significant matters. These two sins, lust and gluttony, are what most people in the West think of when they think of sins. Aquinas, however, cares more about subtler sins, sins that feed on higher human states and can poison all a person's activities.

For him, lust and gluttony work from inclinations that we share with animals, and because of that are both cruder and less likely to pervade the whole personality.

One of these subtler sins is vanity. The vain want to be honored by unworthy people or for unworthy accomplishments. They pursue, for example, the unworthy accomplishment of simply looking beautiful or seek the praise of people whose opinion is of little value. Another subtle sin is anger, and it may differ somewhat from its treatment in Buddhism. Anger is a vice only if it leads people to react violently when they have no justification. If anger is controlled by good judgment, however, it can be a real force for good because it helps animate and sustain a legitimate ethical response. The difference is between the vice of becoming furious at a minor slight and the virtue of using anger to help you do something about a significant injustice, such as when you know someone has been denied employment because of her sex. Virtuous acts involve not simply seeing wrong but doing something about it, and sometimes you need an emotional response like anger to help you to act.

Envy involves resenting the goods—goods like musical talent or fine art, say—that other people possess; it can even involve trying to destroy what is envied. It is one of the most serious vices because it involves failing to love things that are real goods, even if they are goods you do not possess. It is also one of the most mysterious vices because, unlike most other vices, a person gets almost nothing from envy. If I am lustful or gluttonous, I surely get some satisfactions, but all I get from envy is the pain of feeling bad about the good someone else has. That people are envious is one reason many Christians argue that human nature is basically corrupt—that is, that the idea of original sin is true.

Spiritual apathy is called the monk's vice by Aquinas, as it was first recognized in monastic situations and continues to be prevalent in them. It is a failure to pursue the goals that you really want to pursue, a kind of lassitude about seeking the most important things that you want. This vice's character is, I believe, very hard to understand, but I see it in myself and others all the time. That is, you love something good but just cannot bring yourself to do what is necessary to obtain it—for instance, to practice meditation consistently or to write the book you want to write. Spiritual apathy is also a very good example of the way some vices (as well as virtues) can lie so deep within a person that they are never manifested clearly. That is, people who suffer from spiritual apathy may be very active, but their frantic activity covers up the fact that they cannot pursue the goals they most want to obtain.

The last of these vices, avarice or greed, at its simplest level is the pursuit of material goods, the drive to possess objects such as clothes or books. Aquinas thinks, however, it is finally an attempt to protect oneself against the fear produced by the changing character of all things, especially the fear of one's death. That is, one pursues and collects material goods so as not to face the fact that change is constant and death comes to all people. Avarice, then, is a serious attempt to deny the true character of reality.

Pride is a more general sin than any of the preceding seven, although it supports them all. Pride is an inordinate pleasure in and desire for everything having to do with a sense of one's own superiority. It far exceeds the basic respect for one's self that all people should have. For example, it often manifests itself in a self-centered satisfaction with one's natural endowments, and it usually produces a damaging kind of complacency and reliance on one's self. Pride, then, fails to recognize one's vulnerability, one's necessarily limited abilities, and finally one's reliance on God.

Let me now turn to Aquinas' presentation of the virtues. He places them in two groups. In one group are the four cardinal virtues; *cardinal* is derived from the Latin word for "hinge." They are those basic excellencies that everyone needs to live a decent, normal life. Practical wisdom refers to good judgment, judgment that is sensitive to the different kinds of situations we face and that guides our action accordingly. It would tells us, for example, when it is best to be angry and when it is best to forgive. Justice concerns people's relationships with other beings and is especially concerned with being fair to them, with rendering what is due to them. The action itself and not the intent behind it is most important: I should repay the money I owe even if I do not want to repay it.

Courage and moderation largely concern people's relationship with their emotions. Courage overcomes, or corrects, fear in order that we do what we should do. I do not, for instance, let my fear of other people's reactions stop me from challenging racist remarks. Moderation involves harmonizing our desires and emotions, especially our most animal-like desires, so that equanimity and ethical goodness can be maintained. For example, I control my sexual desires so that I can treat as she deserves the attractive but troubled woman I am asked to help. These four virtues are basic to any decent, stable life inside a society and family. They do not necessarily ensure that one will be a great person, but they do help one become at least a good citizen and parent.

The next group of virtues are called infused virtues— infused because they arise from God's direct action. They are religious virtues; that is, they move people beyond ordinary human standards and aspirations, and they involve people being in direct contact with sacred forces. The most important of these are called theological virtues, *theo* being the Greek word for god, and *logical* coming from the Greek word (*logos*) for reason or "thinking about." The three theological virtues are faith, hope, and charity.

Faith is manifested in religious belief, but unlike most intellectual operations that produce belief, faith is animated by love of and contact with God. Faith cannot scientifically prove what it believes, but the assurance that comes from a loving relationship with God underlies the beliefs. Hope's distinguishing mark is a confidence that arises from faith and love's contact with God. Hope enables people to overcome despair but still remain realistic. The hopeful, moreover, recognize their state is due not to their own abilities but to God's power. Aquinas treats both faith and hope in a Christian context, of course, but both refer to modes of living we see in most religions: that is, to kinds of belief and confidence that surpass what people normally have.

Charity is the highest of the theological virtues and underlies both faith and hope. It is close, I think, to true compassion or loving kindness in Buddhism. For Aquinas, this virtue enables a person actually to participate in God's life and therefore to share with God attributes like joy and equanimity. Moreover, charity enables one to see all other beings as creatures like oneself and therefore to recognize that whatever people would want to do for themselves, they should also want to do for all others. It underlies, then, that ability to serve others, and sacrifice for them, that is central to Christianity. Charity is also the ultimate goal that both faith and hope serve. That is, one must believe certain things to be able to be charitable, and one must always have hope, particularly in dark moments, to be able to love.

Your Holiness, we are very interested in your views of what the most significant kinds of vices or virtues are in the Buddhist tradition.

THE BUDDHIST VIEW

DALAI LAMA: This is my perspective. I start from a sense of self, and a sense that I wish for happiness. I wish to be free of suffering, and I am worthy to experience the happiness that I seek, worthy to be free of the suffering. Both the happiness that I strive for, and the suffering that I wish to be free of, are results. Recognizing that, one seeks out the causes that lead to these results: to well-being, or to grief and suffering. One pursues the causes that lead to happiness, and one avoids the causes that lead to suffering and mental afflictions. The vices fall into the latter category, while the virtues fall into the former.

It's within this context that we speak of karma, or actions and their results. The point of karma is not just simply that one shouldn't perform bad deeds, but rather that bad deeds are unwholesome action. One doesn't simply take it at face value, but asks, "Where does this come from, and why is this here?" If you seek the causes that give rise to unwholesome actions, you find mental afflictions. The point is not simply to look at the mental afflictions and say, "Oh, these are bad," and leave it at that; but rather to note that the mental afflictions are results, and to ask, "What are their causes?" You can also ask, "Is it possible to dispel these mental afflictions, and if so, how? What kind of antidote or remedies need to be applied?" And that's where emptiness comes in. Emptiness is the manner in which phenomena arise as dependently related events. It is interrelatedness.

The principal vices, or more accurately, the principal mental afflictions, are attachment and hatred. There are many, many subtle variations of different forms of attachment and hatred, but they all arise principally from these two primary mental afflictions. Now you can ask, "Is there anything more primary than these two?" and the answer is yes. From the Madhyamika Prasangika perspective, we would say the primary mental affliction is the ignorance that grasps onto the inherent existence of phenomena.

Now, let's look at this term *mental affliction.* How is this defined? What are the distinguishing characteristics of mental afflictions? The definition is a mental event that disturbs the equilibrium or peace of the mind. There are, however, wholesome mental events that may make you temporarily unhappy, anxious, or disturbed, but since they are wholesome, they are not mental afflictions.

Compassion is an example of this. In *The Guide to the Bodhisattva Way of Life,* Shantideva points out that when you cultivate compassion, it may be disturbing. It may give rise to anxiety for other sentient beings. He ponders to himself: Isn't it the case that if you cultivate compassion you will feel suffering? And his response is: Yes, but there is a great purpose for cultivating this temporary uneasiness or unhappiness, because of the great benefit that will follow. If we come back then to the definition of mental affliction—a mental factor that disturbs the equilibrium of the mind—we see this is not simply something that temporarily brings about a disturbance, anxiety, or unhappiness. A mental affliction is a mental distortion that not only creates such a disturbance, but in the long run it produces yet further problems. With compassion, there is a temporary disturbance and a long-term benefit.

So, whether or not a mental event creates unhappiness is not the criterion for determining that it is a mental affliction. For example, attachment is a mental affliction, but it may arise simultaneously with a sense of pleasure. Similarly, anger may arise simultaneously with a sense of satisfaction, for example when you've gotten back at someone. A mental event is an affliction if it disturbs the tranquillity of the mind and in the long term creates further problems, continuing disturbances that lead to the perpetuation of unwholesome behavior. If the long-range effects of the mental event are a decrease of problems, then it's not a mental affliction. It may in fact be wholesome.

WHEN FEAR AND ANGER ARE NOT AFFLICTIVE EMOTIONS

DANIEL BROWN: Your Holiness, in my reading of the Abhidharma I have always been puzzled why fear is not on the list of primary and secondary afflictions. In my experience, fear is certainly important.

DALAI LAMA: The reason it not counted in the six primary or twenty secondary delusions is because it is not considered an afflictive emotion. It is not necessarily afflictive. There are virtuous, nonvirtuous, and neutral kinds of fear. For example, fear of evil is itself a virtue. If you are asking why is it not mentioned explicitly among the various mental factors, who knows? There's one Abhidharma text in the Burmese tradition that lists over two hundred different types of mental factors, and fear may be included in that. Do you know of any such elaborate lists in the Theravada tradition?

SHARON SALZBURG: The only instances I know where fear is mentioned are in the sense of moral dread, which is very positive, and in the unwholesome sense of a shrinking aversion.

DALAI LAMA: Fear is one of the things that needs to be overcome to reach enlightenment. The state of fearlessness is something to be attained. But that doesn't prove that it should be counted as one of the afflictive emotions.

DANIEL GOLEMAN: Your Holiness, just as there are different kinds of fear, I wonder about anger. It's on the list of primary afflictions, but is there a virtuous anger? For instance, is anger an evil or a virtue?

DALAI LAMA: Generally speaking, anger is simply something to be rejected. But it is possible that when you look at the motivation for the arising of anger, that motivation may be compassion. So the anger may be a component on your spiritual path, but this is not ordinary anger. In this type of anger, which is aroused by compassion, the mind does indeed become rough, but it has no malice, no intent to give harm. In other words, there is no element of hatred.

DANIEL GOLEMAN: Does it lead to action, an angry act?

DALAI LAMA: Yes, it can lead to forceful or even violent action.

VIRTUOUS VIOLENCE

DANIEL GOLEMAN: So, there can be virtuous violence. Could you give an example?

DALAI LAMA: In the tantric context, there is such a thing as using anger on the path. You see expressions of this in the various wrathful deities. You will find this only in tantra, nowhere else in Buddhism.

DANIEL GOLEMAN: What are wrathful deities angry at? What arouses their anger?

DALAI LAMA: It's difficult to say that they are angry at something, or that they have a clear object that they are angry about. If you want to give a facile answer, you can say simply that they are angry at obstructions, defilements, or inauspicious circumstances. But in terms of the actual practice, there are occasions when an enlightened being seeks to help another sentient being and finds that circumstances do not allow a peaceful approach or engagement. A violent engagement is required in order to serve the sentient being on that occasion, and circumstances induce a wrathful expression.

In cases where logic and reason fail in countering your own negative emotions—in other words, you are not able to talk yourself out of your anger—another antidote is to visualize yourself as a wrathful deity in combat with your own negative emotion. You get angry at your own anger. [*laughs*]

JON KABAT-ZINN: When you generate yourself as a wrathful deity, is there equanimity embedded in it?

DALAI LAMA: When you generate yourself as a wrathful deity, the mind itself is rough. It's not simply a play, putting on a show over perfect equanimity, but in fact there is a corresponding roughness.

COMPASSIONATE ANGER

JON KABAT-ZINN: But is there attachment in the sense that one is lost in the emotion? Does one lose one's wisdom?

DALAI LAMA: Most of the anger that we experience in everyday life is incited by attachment. The kind of anger we are speaking of here is radically different in origin. It is incited by compassion.

JON KABAT-ZINN: And it doesn't bring up or create attachment?

DALAI LAMA: It does not.

ALAN WALLACE: Are the mental afflictions the object of the wrathful deity's anger?

DALAI LAMA: Yes, indeed. In a Buddhist text called the *Four Hundred Verses* by Aryadeva, an Indian pandit, there is a verse which says that the Buddha sees the afflictive emotions as the faults, not the person who possesses them. It's more or less the case that there's no such thing as justified anger directed toward the person. There are no authentic grounds for being angry toward a person.

LEE YEARLEY: Could one's anger toward a quality one thought had to be eliminated lead one to destroy the quality if it might involve destroying the person? For example, as I saw a concentration camp guard in Nazi Germany whose furious hatred was leading him to kill a person, I also realized he was a good father and a person who deserved to live. However, I understood that the only way his hatred could be destroyed was to destroy the person.

DALAI LAMA: This is justified in the following case: You recognize this evil propensity, or vice; you know it must be dispelled because of the ensuing harm that it would bring about; and—this is an extremely important point—out of great compassion arising from the wish to avert the great harm, you see that you must dispel the vice. Recognizing that there is no way to dispel that vice other than through an act of violence, then you may take the life of the person who bears that vice, without ever losing compassion for that person, and while being willing to take on that act yourself.

ROBERT THURMAN: There is a story of the Buddha in an earlier life who killed Devadatta (also in an earlier life) and thereby prevented Devadatta from carrying out his plan of killing 499 people. It was not just the vice but the action he prevented. By killing this one person, he was preventing the murder of 499 others. By preventing the evil of this mass murder, he took upon himself the evil of killing one person.

LEE YEARLEY: And what care must one take when one makes those decisions to see that principle is not misused?

DALAI LAMA: One important factor is that a practitioner must always engage in actions by having two witnesses of the actions: one's own self, and also others. You could come into a situation where there may not be an external witness, but since you are there yourself to witness your act, it calls for a kind of self-honesty. What care should one take to ensure that one has this self-honesty? It would depend on a lot of other factors. Ultimately it comes down to one's own self-discipline, because no matter how elaborate external regulations might be, the human mind is so devious that it would be able to find loopholes. From that point of view, ultimately it depends on the individual. It's very much an individualistic notion of ethics. In fact it combines individualism, perfectionism, and rationalism.

LEE YEARLEY: Does that mean that a person, even an advanced practitioner, should never attempt to kill someone who was going to act destructively just because the practitioner might not be able to honestly evaluate his or her own motives or intentions? Should I say that I must never take a life, because I may find some devious justification that would make it a wrong act?

DALAI LAMA: Two things need to be taken into the balance. On the one hand, something is proscribed, such as killing; on the other hand, it's always a contextual event. That is, one needs to ask: What is the greater need given this circumstance? Something may be proscribed, yet in certain circumstances, the benefit of engaging in it may be greater than the harm created by avoiding it. We find this principle of balance, this give and take, even in the *Vinaya*, [1] the most fundamental Buddhist ethics, and it carries through in the Bodhisattva[2] ethics. One's wisdom is continually called forth to judge the specific circumstances in terms of general principles and the context.

It's quite easy to explain violence in general, but then if we try to implement this injunction against violence, it may be very difficult. Generally, first of all, the motivation is the most important thing, and the result is also important. Violence is just the method, and the method is less important. But the pity is, you don't know the results of your actions until they happen. Violence is like a very strong pill. For a certain illness, it may be very useful, but the side effects are enormous. On a practical level it's very complicated, so it's much safer to avoid acts of violence.

DANIEL GOLEMAN: Your Holiness, you mentioned that motives and results are more important than the methods. How do you distinguish between good and bad motives?

DALAI LAMA: In the case of working for others, the appropriate motive would be the wish to be of benefit to others. However, in the case of one's own self-interest, the appropriate motive would be a wish to attain long-term peace rather than fleeting well-being. There is a pertinent point in the Vinaya literature, which explains the disciplinary codes that monks and nuns must observe to retain the purity of their vows. Take the example of a monk or a nun confronting a situation in which there are only two alternatives: either to take the life of another person, or to take one's own life. Under such circumstances, taking one's life is justified to avoid taking the life of another human being, which would entail transgressing one of the four cardinal vows. Of course, this assumes that one accepts the theory of rebirth; otherwise this is very silly.

ROBERT THURMAN: Your Holiness also mentioned earlier the case of a person who might kill himself, out of compassion, to save someone else from the sin of killing him. This would be a case of killing oneself out of concern for others.

DALAI LAMA: That's an example of the first case, wishing to be of benefit to others. If it's utterly clear that another person plans to kill you, you may take your own life to protect that person from this sin of killing you. In Tibet something comparable took place. Sometimes monks would take their own lives, but not with a gun. They would engage in a certain type of meditation in which their consciousness would be transferred out of their bodies, and they would die. They would do this to protect other people from killing them.

CLIFF SARON: But the motivation to kill was total in the person who was about to murder you. Doesn't that have consequence?

DALAI LAMA: This goes into the complexities of karma. For the karma of an action to be complete, there has to be a basis for the act of killing, namely the being to be killed; there has to be the intention; there has to be a preparation; and there has to be the completion of the act. In this case, the basis and the intention are there; the preparation might even be there; but at least you're protecting the person from one or two of those four, which means the karmic results will be less. But it's not as if that person completely escapes the consequences. There are cases in which you can accumulate the karma for something without actually committing the act. That is, you can accumulate an act without committing it. In other cases it is possible to commit an act without accumulating it. For example, if you walk along a path and you unintentionally step on an insect, you have committed the act of killing, but, ethically speaking, you have not accumulated it. Also in terms of the intention for a negative act, you need three factors. First, there has to be a mental affliction activated in the process. Second, there has to be a motive, and third, there needs to be a recognition of the object.

ROBERT LIVINGSTON: Let's take the case of the dropping of the bombs on Japan. The people who did that were told that they would save a million lives.

DANIEL GOLEMAN: Was that a Bodhisattva act?

DALAI LAMA: It's very difficult to judge. Theoretically speaking, yes, it's a possibility, if it was done in order to save a lot of human lives.

ROBERT THURMAN: Your Holiness, isn't it the case that when a Bodhisattva does such a thing, it's highly exceptional? The Bodhisattva virtually always tries not to commit any violence. A person almost has to be clairvoyant really to judge the consequences. That's why only an advanced Bodhisattva can drop a bomb, but that would paralyze most people from performing such an exceptional act. I don't think that Harry Truman was a Bodhisattva! [laughter]

LEE YEARLEY: In Christian theology, there is the notion of a sin of omission. By omitting to do something that prevents a death, you yourself are guilty of that death. Suppose Harry Truman had decided that he ought not to drop the bomb because he wasn't clairvoyant, because he doubted his own judgment and didn't feel he had enough information. Would he then be guilty for those lives that were lost because he failed to believe in his own ability to judge?

DALAI LAMA: In the case of a person who sees somebody drowning and says, "It's not my business," and walks away, there is an omission, a non-act. And we can ask whether that has negative karmic consequences. That's a simple case; later we can go to a more difficult case.

LEE YEARLEY: If you saw someone drowning and thought, "It's not my business," that's such a clear violation of a sense of connectedness or relationship to others that it is just a vicious act.

I'm thinking of a situation where you doubt that you understand well enough what the consequences may be. For example, you see someone striking a small child rather viciously, but you don't know if perhaps there are good reasons for this person's action. If you don't act to stop it, and it turns out that you have not intervened where you clearly should have because there was an act of violence, are you responsible for not trusting your immediate judgment that violence was being done because you doubted that you knew enough about what was involved?

DALAI LAMA: In such circumstances, it would depend very much on that person's attitude in confronting such a situation. If he turned away from the child who is being beaten simply to avoid getting involved in others' affairs, he would have a problem. On the other hand, he might have been motivated to turn away from the situation because his involvement might have increased the person's anger and the child might suffer more. So it depends very much on what kind of motivation or attitude you have at that moment. Coming back to your issue, Bob, of dropping the bombs on Nagasaki and Hiroshima: We can't judge this act ethically only by the particular moment in history. We have to look at the long-term consequences, and if we do so, specifically in terms of the immense proliferation of nuclear weapons, then we can be unequivocal in declaring that as an unethical act. Even in those particular circumstances there may have been some positive motivation, but since then, it has definitely created a lot of negative consequences. Much more fear has been brought about due to that.

Social Ethics

ROBERT THURMAN: It seems to me that the discussion has largely revolved around the individual's conscience and behavior and the impact of institutional forces, governmental and religious, on that behavior. I would like to turn to an issue that we all face, that certain nations, collective governments, have been able to create weapons of mass destruction. Some of the servants who contribute to that are nominally ethical persons, who believe in contributing to the welfare of the group, but have somehow made possible this threat to the whole world. How do you and His Holiness meet that issue?

LEE YEARLEY: I think one of the most chastening and most distressing things about the modern world is the growth of nation states and what nation states have meant. Winston Churchill said that the wars that democracies fight will be the most horrible wars that humans have ever fought. I think he was right. It has to do with seeing this collective, this group, this nation, as something that must be protected at all costs, that people must contribute to and sacrifice for. Somehow, marshaling all the participants in the group for a common purpose makes them almost demonic entities. I think we have cases in American history where the nation America has done things that almost no individual or group of individuals in America would ever do. What you do about it other than the very weak notion of being aware of it, I'm not sure.

Dalai Lama: Perhaps there is a parallel with your story of someone keeping the gun, and believing that the right thing to do is to give it back when asked. Instead of a gun, we have nuclear armaments in vast proportions.

Jon Kabat-Zinn: It really hinges on the critical point that societies on the planet may be moving in the direction of autodestruction on a very massive scale, killing not just one small part of the self but the whole world, which would of course select against any further development. You could make an analogy to autoimmune disease, where the body does not recognize its true nature and kills itself; in the same way, the small-minded rationalist or the impassioned perfectionist could wind up being so toxic on a global level that it kills the entire organism. So, the real question at the moment is whether, by invoking a transcendent intelligence or emergent properties of intelligence within the brain and the nervous system, we can individually and collectively come to an awareness of this problem that will allow us to avoid destruction. Is there a way out of the dilemma that is biologically valid?

A monk: The destruction that faces the human race now seems to depend largely on the fact that science, at least applied science, seems to be free of values, without any ethical foundation. Must that be so? Is that necessarily part of the correct functioning and progress of science?

Francisco Varela: I don't agree that science is free of values. It is not separate from the social life of a country or of the globe. Decisions about whether a weapon gets built or a particular technological device gets installed, and then trashes the environment, are always political, moral, historical, and economic decisions that involve the entire society. The values of applied science are the values of that society in which the application takes place. You cannot centrifugate science as a separate component. When a doctor in a clinic decides whether or not to terminate a patient's life support, that's a technological decision, but it is based on a whole host of positions that are inseparably social. The ethics that we are talking about here apply everywhere, science included, and it seems to distort the whole nature of the scientific process to try to set it apart as if it were in the attic, rather than in the kitchen with everybody else.

LEE YEARLEY: I think that's largely true, but it's also too easy, because it assumes that scientists would be heroic not to pursue a line of research that may be used destructively. But given the fact that we reward scientists in various ways, and that there should at least be an ethic to the profession, I think we have a right to ask them to refrain from doing something if they believe it is likely to lead to bad results.

FRANCISCO VARELA: Historically that has never happened. It will only happen when it becomes a socially negative act to pursue, and when you don't provide the means to pursue it with grants and positions and prizes. If you leave it to the individual it doesn't work, first of all because scientists are as confused about ethics as anybody else, and second because a scientist does not work just because he or she wants to. The scientist needs the means, and high technology requires money and infrastructural support, so we're back to the same point. We cannot dump the decision whether or not to pursue a certain technology on the back of one group of people. That's far too optimistic, and it fails.

LEE YEARLEY: I don't want to say that it is simply the scientist's responsibility and that the scientist is not part of a society. I do say that sometimes you have to make very dramatic decisions that may hurt you a good deal. Scientists sometimes are in those positions. It may in fact involve something far beyond the normal to do it, which is why I called it heroic, but I think at times we have a right to ask that of people, and to judge them if they fail to do it.

Notes

1. *Vinaya* is the portion of the Buddhist canon that deals with monastic discipline and ethics in general.

2. A Bodhisattva is a spiritually advanced person who is fulfilling a vow to benefit all sentient beings.

9

The Roots of Self-Esteem

DIFFERENCES EAST AND WEST

LANGUAGE AND CULTURE shape how we interpret and define emotion. For example, the feeling of *yugan*— roughly, an aesthetic moment of oneness—in Japan, or *rasa*, a wordless appreciation in India, have no exact counterparts in English. Similarly, Tibetan has no word for the English term *emotion*. And, although it is central to the Tibetan concept of well-being, the concept of equanimity is not included as a major emotional state in English. A great many Tibetan terms that refer to subtle aspects of meditation and consciousness have no equivalent in English. Emotions are experienced through the lens of culture.

The framing question of this discussion on emotion is whether historical and cultural conditions might give rise to new emotions or their expression. The case in point is self-esteem: the Dalai Lama is astounded to hear that many Westerners suffer from feelings of low self-esteem. There is no such concept of self-loathing or self-deprecation—or, as the Dalai Lama puts it, "a lack of compassion for oneself" or "self-directed contempt"—in Tibetan culture. This leads to a wide-ranging exploration of the root of this condition, the difference between a feeling of "emptiness" in the psychological sense of inadequacy and the realization of emptiness in Buddhist practice, which—along with the cultivation of loving kindess toward oneself—the Dalai Lama suggests might be an antidote for feelings of low self-esteem and a basis for genuine self-acceptance.

LEE YEARLEY: Your Holiness, do you think emotions are in part products of history? Some philosophers have argued that because Westerners live a far richer, more complicated emotional life than ever before, a more precise set of terms has entered our vocabulary, terms such as callow, diffident, mawkish, shy, put-upon.

ALAN WALLACE: These terms cannot easily be translated.

DALAI LAMA: It can happen historically that unprecedented circumstances elicit unprecedented emotions. It's also possible that previous emotions may vanish as the external circumstances change.

LEE YEARLEY: What would be some examples?

DALAI LAMA: For example, in a materially affluent society, a great deal of competition can arise over acquiring material goods, which then leads to a great deal of anxiety. This might be a case of unprecedented emotions created by the circumstances. Another example, prior to the present Gulf crisis, a certain type of emotional response was aroused at the mention of Iraq. Now the situation is changed, and when someone says Iraq, another whole set of emotions is aroused.

DANIEL GOLEMAN: But those particular feelings were possible before. You have only applied them to a new object. Are there new kinds of feelings that people now have that didn't exist in a previous time?

DALAI LAMA: It's possible that if a new kind of object were created, it could elicit unprecedented emotions. That object might be a whole circumstance or environment. Fundamentally, craving and aversion are ever present, and it's doubtful that a new class of distinctions can be historically created in humanity.

LEE YEARLEY: Let me give you an example of what I mean. Extensive research has been done concerning the rise of nineteenth-century French novelists such as Flaubert. After this literature has become part of people's lives, their diaries and actions reveal a very different set of problems, terms, and ideas about emotions arising. It's difficult to trace what caused what, but it seems that a literary depiction of a set of difficulties that could arise between a man and a woman began to create those difficulties and, therefore, created new emotions between men and women.

DANIEL BROWN: When we talked earlier about emotions, there was a rather simple list of emotional facial display patterns. However, we know from experience that there are many more types and subtle nuances of emotions than were listed. There aren't a lot of variations in the facial display muscles or in the autonomic or visceral response. Since the physiology is rather simple, it has been suggested that thought or language helps give the specificity to emotions. So the question is, can the development of a new language, as in the novel, create new specificity or subtleties in emotions?

ROBERT THURMAN: The new concepts and modes of interpretation are really just adding complexity to the same basic emotion. The Buddhist literature, especially from India, from ancient times has a very complex analysis of emotion. It's questionable whether any really new emotion has come up, although certainly new modes might arise.

DALAI LAMA: It's certainly the case that our usage of language can enhance or increase certain mental distortions, but whether it can actually freshly create new types of distortions or emotions is an open question.

FRANCISCO VARELA: It does seem possible. For example, in Spanish literature, a particular way of relating self to others appears in the novels of the eighteenth century that did not exist before. A new word, *verguenza ajena*, appears in the language for the shame that one feels on someone else's behalf when they are doing something that is embarrassing for them. It's not ordinary embarrassment, because we are not the actors, and it's not pity, since we recognize in ourselves the other's lack of skill.

DALAI LAMA: Still, there is a recognition of the other as another human being?

FRANCISCO VARELA: Sure, but that person doesn't have to be related to you, or a personal friend.

DALAI LAMA: There is always a relationship in a universal sense. I relate to that person as a human being. I understand that at some point in the past, 1 or 2 million years ago, the human brain was smaller than it is now. In the evolution of the human brain, was there also a change in size of the front and back parts of the brain relative to each other?

FRANCISCO VARELA: Yes.

DALAI LAMA: Does that lead us to believe that the capacity for emotions also changed?

DANIEL GOLEMAN: The part of the brain that controls emotion is very ancient. It's called the reptilian brain because we share it with reptiles. What was added in evolution was the cortex, the thinking brain and the ability to have subtle emotions. An alligator can apparently have fear or anger, just as we can, but more subtle distinctions came with the cortex. The complex and subtle feelings we are discussing now happened only very late in evolution.

EMOTIONAL DEVELOPMENT DURING CHILDHOOD

DALAI LAMA: Leaving aside history, just take the case of one person's human development. Does a young child who has not been educated have fewer sorts of emotions than a well-educated child?

DANIEL GOLEMAN: Yes. As a child grows, there are specific stages at which certain emotions emerge. For instance, social emotions such as embarrassment and shame typically don't emerge until around the age of five or so. Even in the first three or four years of life, different emotions emerge as different parts of the brain fully mature.

DANIEL BROWN: The earliest ones are happiness, sadness, anger, and fear. Then it gets more complex. Certain emotions that involve a lot of cognition, like guilt, come much later.

DALAI LAMA: Is there any distinction in terms of whether the child is raised in religion or not?

DANIEL BROWN: No. It's universal.

DALAI LAMA: Among adults, is there any distinction between religious and nonreligious people in terms of the variety of their emotions?

FRANCISCO VARELA: That hasn't been studied. It is clear that the vocabulary referring to emotions in different languages can vary dramatically.

DANIEL BROWN: And we also know that in some cultural groups, certain emotions are more evident than in other cultural groups. For example, expressions of anger are much less evident in Japanese culture. Contempt is more evident in French culture than in American culture.

DANIEL GOLEMAN: When Paul Ekman, who did facial studies on universal emotions, went to Japan, he found that people watching distressing films showed very little emotion, except when they thought they were alone. He used a hidden camera and had people watch a movie. Alone, they freely showed the same emotions in Japan as in everywhere else in the world. But when one other person of authority was in the room, they showed no emotion. So the facial expression of emotion is affected by culture, but the feelings are there.

NEGATIVE SELF-APPRAISALS

SHARON SALZBERG: Lee talked earlier about a strong belief among some Westerners that evil lies at the very center of a human being. This seems very different from the Buddhist understanding that the natural state of the mind is radiant and pure, and that the defilements that create so much suffering only visit us, and are not inherent in the mind. I would like to ask you about the mind state, very common in Westerners, of strong hatred toward oneself. In Theravadin Buddhism, we teach that the strongest cause for loving kindness, or *metta*, is to see the goodness in somebody, but very often people say they cannot see their own goodness. Or, when we ask people to reflect on good things they have done in the past so that the mind is filled with joy, self-respect, and confidence, they say they cannot easily do this. They can dwell on the bad things they have done, but not on the good. When we talk about generosity, they say they are already generous, but only because they feel they themselves don't deserve to have what they are giving away. Because people so often express that they can feel love and compassion for other beings more easily than for themselves, what does it mean to teach sacrificing oneself for others? For these people, the emphasis on self-sacrifice is often seen not as true loving kindness, but simply as more self-contempt and unworthiness. Sometimes, Your Holiness, there's another component as well. It's not just that people wish to be happy and aren't. They wish to be happy but feel they don't deserve to be; they feel guilty, as if it would somehow be wrong for them to be happy. So when we teach loving kindess and compassion, should we talk very specifically about loving yourself?

[After a long exchange in Tibetan, Alan Wallace comments that this concept is alien to His Holiness.]

DALAI LAMA: Is this self-contempt or lack of compassion for oneself something that arises now and then as a result of specific circumstances, or is it a matter of temperament, an enduring mental trait?

SHARON SALZBERG: I think this is an enduring mental trait that is very commonly found in Western culture.

DANIEL BROWN: Cognitive therapists have discovered that many ordinary people carry on an incessant and very negative inner monologue. They say to themselves in effect, "I can't do this. I hate myself. Nothing good will ever happen." This becomes a constant habit, even when people aren't aware of it. Therapists say you have to intervene and intentionally think positive thoughts as an antidote to change this habit, which is very difficult. When people get depressed, this negative talk becomes much more intense. It's also very characteristic that when Westerners start to look inward, in psychotherapy or in meditation, a lot of this self-hatred emerges in their early experiences.

JON KABAT-ZINN: Your Holiness, this problem of low self-esteem is very common in the West. People ordinarily are not even aware of the negative inner monologue. Much of this comes from early childhood experiences: a mother is angry and says to a child, "You're a bad girl," where what she really means is, "I don't like what you're doing." The message, "I'm bad," stays with the child even when she has grown and forgotten why. We see this in almost everybody who comes to the hospital with medical problems. People don't feel like they're worth much.

DALAI LAMA: Are those people violent?

JON KABAT-ZINN: No, they are normal, ordinary people.

SHARON SALZBERG: That's us. [*laughter*]

DALAI LAMA: If people with such low self-esteem are caught in a situation where they lose their temper, don't they have a strong feeling that their own self is worth defending?

JON KABAT-ZINN: Sometimes they just give up. They feel helpless, as if they deserve whatever bad happens. On the other hand, many people respond to deep inner feelings of low self-esteem by creating aggression. They run over others like steam rollers. Deep down, they are uncomfortable with themselves and don't want to look at it, so instead they project outward power. That very easily leads to aggression, violence, and lack of sympathy for others' feelings. This is a very big problem in the West.

DANIEL BROWN: Usually it doesn't lead to aggression or violence directed outwardly, but to more negative self-hatred.

DALAI LAMA: What do you as healers find is beneficial to help such people? What methods are effective?

JON KABAT-ZINN: We find that training people in meditation, particularly mindfulness meditation, is very effective. If you ask people who know nothing about meditation to sit very still and watch their breathing, the first thing they notice is that it's difficult because thoughts come and go. If you then ask the people to watch the content of the thought, but not get drawn into it, they observe that a thought comes up such as, "I am no good." Before they thought that was the truth; now they see it's just a thought. As they go back to the breathing and the thought passes, they feel a sense of liberation. Even in people with serious problems like chronic pain or heart disease, a change in the way they see themselves can happen quite rapidly, although the problem doesn't go away immediately. Often after as little as eight or ten weeks, people begin catching themselves, not during meditation, but in daily life. When you feel bad about yourself, other people, or a social situation, you recognize this as a thought, not as the truth, and then you let go of it. You have a much greater sense of inner balance and not such a problem with low self-esteem.

SHARON SALZBERG: It also helps to offer teachings about morality so that people can respect themselves for leading a more virtuous life. Also, when we teach loving kindness meditation, it's important that people include themselves in the loving feeling and not just other beings.

JON KABAT-ZINN: Are you surprised?

DALAI LAMA: Oh, yes, very much. I thought I had a very good acquaintance with the mind, but now I feel quite ignorant. I find this very, very strange, and I wonder where it comes from. Are you all suffering from nervous disorders, and is the source of such self-deprecation simply physiological?

CAUSES OF LOW SELF-ESTEEM

THUBTEN JINPA: Maybe it really comes from your culture, maybe your religious heritage, and these kind of social factors.

DALAI LAMA: Perhaps it arises from an absolutist mentality. That is, if something is somewhat negative then one labels it as absolutely negative; and if something is rather good, it is seen as absolutely good, ignoring all the subtle variations in between. That might give rise to this mental dysfunction.

JON KABAT-ZINN: There is another possibility here, though they're not mutually exclusive. It's related to what Dan Goleman was saying earlier about people feeling that they have no control of their lives. In our society in the past, there were many systems that gave the individual a sense of belonging and connectedness. The systems provided some control and defined a little world that made sense. The church and the extended family, for instance, were very powerful forces in people's lives. Nowadays, the church in the West is much weaker and less important to many people. The family has very often broken up. Work also is very fragmented: it's no longer the farm that your father had, and your father's father, and on back in time on the same land. Social relationships now are much more in flux, and this makes it difficult for young people to know where they belong in the society.

LEE YEARLEY: It isn't just a modern phenomenon. When Alexis de Tocqueville observed America in 1830, he identified one of the two major characteristics of Americans as what he called "American nervousness." Although he was in favor of a liberal, democratic society, he thought the price for such a society was quite extraordinary; because of it, you couldn't place yourself. Not being clear who you were, or what was valuable, seemed built into the system. He believed that the American experiment might therefore fail, and this was close to two hundred years ago.

DALAI LAMA: Does a high percentage of the American population have this type of attitude?

JON KABAT-ZINN: Very high.

DALAI LAMA: Is there much difference for Europeans or South Americans?

FRANCISCO VARELA: It's very much less common, Your Holiness. I think part of the reason is something that was mentioned earlier: the possibility that emotions are partly culturally conditioned by language. When I go to the United States, the enormous amount of talk about self-esteem surprises me. In Europe and South America, that is much less the case. In France, for example, the word for self-esteem is not normally heard. The language reinforces the emotion and makes it very prominent in their lives. I think it might be a very good example of how history, culture, and language shape a certain repertoire of emotions.

JON KABAT-ZINN: It may be possible, as we were saying earlier, to have a new emotion that didn't exist five hundred years ago. This may be one we have discovered ourselves.

LEE YEARLEY: One reason for this is the very prominent religious notion of a God who judges.

A MONK: The concept of original sin reinforces this. I've also met quite a few people for whom the Buddhist doctrine of no truly existent self reinforces their low self-esteem.

LEE YEARLEY: It is sometimes said of American Christians that their Christianity only goes as far as the crucifixion, and they forget everything else that happened. In the fuller Christian story, Jesus is killed, but arises again to make the community live in a particular way. But they only see that goodness is destroyed, they don't see how it continues to live, so one side of the picture is left out completely.

DALAI LAMA: Does this mentality occur among mute people?

DANIEL GOLEMAN: Yes, Your Holiness. In fact, in America people with handicaps often have it even more.

DALAI LAMA: I mean, are there such obstructions for people who have no possibility of communicating in words?

FRANCISCO VARELA: There is the case of Helen Keller, who was born blind and deaf. However, she had a very good tutor, who communicated through touch. She eventually learned to read and write, and described her experience of being blind and deaf. Her description is not a socialized image of a self, but a very different kind of self which then became socialized when she learned to communicate within the culture. It is a perfect example of what you're asking, and the answer would be definitely yes, the lack of language in participation in a culture would shape the sense of self.

DALAI LAMA: An important term in Tibetan Buddhism is *self-centeredness*, which means cherishing your own well-being above that of anybody else. Is it possible to have self-centeredness simultaneously with this lack of self-esteem?

DANIEL BROWN: Yes, they often go together. People with extreme esteem problems often have a puffed-up, grandiose self-image, as well as low self-esteem.

DALAI LAMA: These people with low self-esteem certainly have a sense of "I." Don't they also have some sense that they want to be happy?

DANIEL BROWN: Yes, of course, very strongly.

DANIEL GOLEMAN: Wanting to be happy is self-centeredness?

DALAI LAMA: In Tibetan Buddhism one can ask, "Does a buddha have self-interest or only concern for other people?" The answer—and this is a crucial point—is that a buddha has both. Similarly a Bodhisattva, who is free of self-centeredness, still wishes to attain full enlightenment for the benefit of all creatures; and so such a person has both self-interest as well as public interest. Without that, there'd be no confidence and you'd have very low self-esteem. But self-centeredness is something beyond that, and a buddha or a Bodhisattva does not have self-centeredness. Self-centeredness wishes for one's own happiness but discards the well-being of others. It doesn't need to be grandiose, but it does make oneself the priority and put everything else second.

DANIEL BROWN: There has been a lot of study in Western psychotherapy of people who have narcissistic personality disorders, which are extreme versions of self-esteem problems. They usually have very low self-esteem, as well as grandiosity. Some start with a complaint about their own low self-esteem and through psychotherapy discover a more grandiose self-image, so that eventually they develop a more balanced view of themselves. Others start very puffed up, and over time, in psychotherapy, they uncover their low self-esteem. Again, the successful outcome in psychotherapy is a more balanced view of themselves.

We also find that people who are narcissistic or have chronic self-esteem problems have difficulty holding the self and the other in their awareness at the same time. For example, narcissistic clients come into psychotherapy so filled up with themselves that they're not aware of the therapist. They fill the entire room, and the therapist gets bored because he or she doesn't feel present for the patient. Sometimes the opposite is true; the patient will be so taken by the presence of the therapist, idealize him or her, or see the therapist as very powerful, that the patient's sense of self is lost in the presence of the therapist. People with these extreme narcissistic disorders can't keep the self and the other together in their awareness at the same time, so they alternate between all self and

196   *Emotion and Culture*

no other, or all other and no self. This is part of the problem
that needs to be corrected.

DALAI LAMA: In these cases of people with low self-
esteem, three things seem to be present. First, they certainly
have a sense of self; secondly, they do want to be happy; but
thirdly, there is this self-directed contempt, or anger. This
may also be related to hopelessness and despair. You com-
mented that when people with these kind of problems are
taught through mindfulness meditation to watch their
thoughts arising, and they realize that they are mere
thoughts, this somehow helps reduce their low self-esteem. Is
this because by so doing, they feel a sense of achievement? Is
that what reduces their low self-esteem, or is it something
else?

THE ABILITY TO MAKE THINGS HAPPEN

JON KABAT-ZINN: I think it's something else as well,
but you've put your finger on a very important point in this
extreme form of discouragement. Self-efficacy has been the
subject of much research in Western psychology in the past
fifteen years. The belief in one's ability to make something
happen in a certain domain can be very specific. If you do not
believe in your ability to stop smoking, we can predict that
you will not be able to stop smoking very easily. Take fixing
a car: some people look under the hood and say, "My God, I
could never do that." They will never fix a car. Other people
say, "Well, I don't know, but let's try." They are much happier and better adjusted, and they also recover much more
quickly from diseases. This belief in one's own competence is
the strongest predictor for change in patients who are recovering from heart disease and arthritis, and it actually correlates with certain measures of the immune system.

To answer your question more specifically, it increases people's feelings of self-efficacy when they discover in meditation
that they do not have to feel weighed down by a thought—

when they recognize the thought "I'm no good" as a thought rather than as true, and let it go. The next time it happens, they let it come, catch it, and then let it go, so they don't feel so depressed. Their belief in their capacity to become more skillful grows, and that feeling of mastery is a very positive way to increase self-esteem.

DALAI LAMA: Do you apply other methods, such as giving people with low self-esteem a certain task, watching them perform it, praising them when they do it well, and in that way boosting their morale or self-esteem?

JON KABAT-ZINN: Yes, of course it helps.

METHODS FOR MANAGING LOW SELF-ESTEEM

DANIEL BROWN: Let me speak to the issue of methods here. Jon has talked about using meditation to handle this; we'd like to see it done more, but this approach is unique to his own work. In the West, the usual approach to these kinds of problems is psychotherapy, and within psychotherapy there are two methods that have been useful for this problem. One method, cognitive therapy, works directly with the thoughts. You first identify the pattern of negative thinking, for example, by asking people to write a list of their typical negative thoughts, such as, "I'm a bad person; I can't do anything; bad things will always happen; it's going to get worse." Then, on the other side of the page they write down the positive thought, or affirmation, that serves as an antidote. For example, in opposition to "It's going to get worse," people write, "Take one step at a time," or they counter the statement "I'm a bad person" by saying what they value about themselves.

They then take those affirmations and practice holding them in their mind continuously, like a meditation or a mantra. It's been found that when people practice those affirmations regularly, twenty minutes or half an hour a day, or a few minutes at times interspersed throughout the day, this whole pattern of negative thinking eventually changes, and they think more positively about themselves. So that's one way: identifying the negative and applying the antidote, which is affirmation.

DALAI LAMA: So it's almost like reminding oneself of one's own value and worth.

DANIEL BROWN: Yes. Your Holiness, I understand that you have a similar practice in your tradition that has to do with applying an opposite as the antidote to negative behavior. This is very similar except it applies to thought rather than behavior. If you have bad thoughts, you apply good thoughts as the antidote.

A second approach used in psychotherapy has more to do with the quality of the relationship between people, in this case between the patient and the therapist. It's believed that a patient who thinks so negatively was ignored by parents and others while growing up, or was not praised enough for realistic accomplishments. These people have a legitimate need in their desire to be admired. So the therapist tries to praise them for realistic accomplishments. Over time, if the therapist is continuously interested, respectful, and admiring of the patient, the self-hatred will change and the person will develop a more healthy, balanced sense of themselves. It's as if they're being re-parented by the therapist.

DALAI LAMA: I am trying to trace the etiology, the natural causal links leading to this. To trace this, we note there is a sense of self that wishes for one's own happiness, and then the low self-esteem and self-deprecation come in. But underlying this, might there not already be compassion toward oneself on a deeper level? In that case, the low self-esteem is a distortion on a more superficial level, whereas underlying that is a sense of appropriate self-love.

JON KABAT-ZINN: I think that's true, but if you can't get in touch with that sense of self-love then you feel cut off and alone.

DALAI LAMA: If there is no genuine sense of love underlying all that emotion, then even if others praise you, you
are not affected by that praise. When others praise a person
with low self-esteem, he or she says they're wrong. The
method that Dan Brown described about affirmations to
counter negative feelings was almost like reminding the patients of their own value. When the patients read the list of
negative words on one side, and positive words on the other,
it reminds them that they can do something, they actually are
worthy in these ways, and it seems to help them. But unless
one assumes there is some kind of self-love underlying their
emotion, it would be difficult to understand; there would be
no motivation.

JON KABAT-ZINN: I think there are deep reservoirs
of love underlying all human beings.

DALAI LAMA: Oh, yes. I believe that's human nature.
So long as one is a human being, that self-love should be
there.

JON KABAT-ZINN: Your Holiness, you're absolutely
right. For instance, many people have trouble with their bodies. They don't like their body, they feel it's too this, too much
that, not beautiful enough, whatever. When therapy is successful, or when people have positive experiences in meditation, they are clearing the channel to the deeper sense of well-
being inside.

DALAI LAMA: This is what Tibetan yogis are trying to
do through their meditation, so without trying, they've already achieved that! [laughter]

JON KABAT-ZINN: When people start to pay attention in the moment to their bodies, they very often discover
that underneath the surface dislike, they accept their bodies.
But the surface thoughts going on all the time are very
strongly negative, so it prevents them from getting in touch
with the deeper feeling of wholeness. If everybody, all 5 billion people on the planet, has this connectedness, this love

and clarity under the surface, then the key question is, particularly for those who have very strong problems with this, how to get in touch with that peace and love inside oneself most effectively and reliably, and in a way that leads to long-lasting profound understanding.

CULTIVATING LOVINGKINDNESS
TOWARD ONESELF

DALAI LAMA: I think one Buddhist principle which has a strong relevance to this whole issue is the assertion that the Buddha nature is something that pervades all sentient beings. When you apply that personally, it follows that the essential nature of your own mind is utterly pure; and this provides a basis for self-confidence and also for overcoming despair.

JON KABAT-ZINN: But it requires belief, and you said that 4 billion people on the planet don't have belief.

DALAI LAMA: One doesn't start off with the assertion of Buddha nature, because that would simply be a leap of faith. Rather, one first seeks the realization of emptiness. So there are two avenues: for some people, belief will be the initial step, but there is another avenue that is not simply belief, but the pursuit of the realization of emptiness. On the basis of that realization, one can see that mental distortions are purely adventitious. They're not intrinsic to the nature of the mind, and one can therefore be freed of them. Now you can introduce the assertion of the buddha nature, and it has a very solid foundation, not simply an assertion of a belief.

JON KABAT-ZINN: This could be a real problem in America if you use the wrong words, because what you mean by emptiness is very, very different from what Westerners understand. They already feel totally empty! [*laughter*]

DALAI LAMA: Westerners' conception of emptiness is thoroughly empty! This Western notion, which is a false conception of emptiness, is that it's just empty, whereas the right conception of emptiness is that it's thoroughly full. Normally when we use the term *ego*, or self-identity, there may be two connotations, one which is negative and one which need not be negative. One sense of self-identity is negative in the sense that it arises from self-importance, arrogance, and so on, without any valid basis. That kind of a strong sense of self-identity is false. But there could be another sense of self-identity, or ego, which, in fact, would be stronger in Bodhisattvas than in ordinary people; for Bodhisattvas are beings who are prepared to sacrifice their own welfare for the benefit of others. In place of their own welfare, they cherish the well-being of other sentient beings. To achieve that strength of will, you need first of all a strong sense of self-identity, and on that basis you can switch your priorities from self to others. Thus, the Bodhisattvas' sense of self-identity is even stronger than that of an ordinary person who is not able to sacrifice his or her own welfare for the sake of others. For this, you need extraordinary willpower, and you develop that with strong self-confidence.

JON KABAT-ZINN: This is relevant to what Lee Yearley described concerning the sin of spiritual apathy, which is a widespread problem in this society. I wonder whether this could be connected with the whole question of developing a strong sense of determination, but without the negative egotistic connotations.

DANIEL BROWN: In Western psychotherapy, we have a concept called healthy self-esteem, which is different from what you're describing about Bodhisattvas, Your Holiness. An individual with healthy self-esteem is not grandiose, not arrogant without basis, but most important is that the person maintains self-esteem relatively independent from the context. For the ordinary person with low self-esteem, self-value depends on context. For example, I worry about how other people see me, and I need a certain kind of admiration or praise. If other people criticize me, my self-esteem is lower. I'm dependent on how other people view me for my sense of

my own worth. Or, my self-worth may depend on my own
evaluation of my accomplishments. If I do something good, I
feel puffed up; if I fall short of my personal standards, then I
feel bad. People with healthy self-esteem are less dependent
both on the external context and on the discrepancy between
their performance at the moment and their own internal standards for that performance. So we can say their self-esteem is
steady, without a lot of change.

DALAI LAMA: Because it's based on evidence, based
on reason, then it has a greater stability.

DANIEL BROWN: Yes, it has greater stability, so these
people are not easily affected by whether others think badly
of them or admire them greatly. It's beyond praise or blame
in that sense, and it's less affected by whether what they're
doing at any given time falls short of their own internal standards or goals. What's missing in this Western notion of
healthy self-esteem is the very thing that your tradition emphasizes. The concept of healthy self-esteem usually emphasizes autonomy, that is, independence. The concept of the
Bodhisattva emphasizes relationship to others, doing things
for others, and in that sense it seems different.

DALAI LAMA: I gave the example of a Bodhisattva,
but this has a much broader relevance.
I spoke about this issue of a proper, or healthy, self-identity
with reference to the Bodhisattva because one usually associ-
ates a Bodhisattva with self-sacrifice. Nevertheless, a strong
sense of self-identity can be relevant to many people who are
not Bodhisattvas. To have such a strong and authentic sense
of self, one doesn't necessarily have to have a deep sense of
altruism, cherishing others deeply. Not only Bodhisattvas,
but practitioners such as *shravakas*[1] and *pratyekabuddhas*.[2]
certainly have a strong sense of "I" who shall refrain from
unwholesome actions. So they too have a strong sense of personal identity.

GENUINE SELF-ACCEPTANCE

DANIEL GOLEMAN: What are the qualities or traits of mind of this kind of identity? What mental factors would be dominant in the mind of such a person?

DALAI LAMA: This proper sense of a strong self-identity, or self-confidence, is not something that would arise in dependence on just one cause, but is due to many causes. For example, according to Buddhist psychology, self-confidence may arise without conceit or pride, and on the basis of self-confidence one might aspire for something, but without craving. Similarly, one might have compassion without afflictive attachment associated with it. One distinguishes among the different kinds of self-confidence by the means of discriminating intelligence.

ALAN WALLACE: The term we're translating here as self-confidence or self-esteem also carries the meaning of conscience, both personal and public. The distinction between personal and public conscience is that the first operates even when you're in solitude: your conscience, or self-esteem, will not allow you to engage in certain unwholesome actions because you think it's beneath you, or it's inappropriate, regardless of whether anybody ever finds out. Public conscience involves taking others' awareness of you into account. Both of these are regarded as wholesome states of mind. One can have both of these very strongly, without any sense of self-effacement, lack of self-esteem, or despair.

DANIEL BROWN: That definition emphasizes restraint from unwholesome action. Does that also include unwholesome thought?

ALAN WALLACE: Oh, yes: body, speech, and mind.

THUBTEN JINPA: There's a sense of caution, but without discouragement.

DALAI LAMA: Language does create some difficulties. Perhaps eventually we can come up with one universal language. It would save a lot of time! [*laughter*]

For people who have such a problem and are not Buddhists, what is the best method?

DANIEL GOLEMAN: Cognitive therapy.

DALAI LAMA: Can you take elements from Buddhism and apply them for people who don't believe?

DANIEL GOLEMAN: A very important part of cognitive therapy is mindfulness, just learning to notice that you have these thoughts.

ALEX BERZIN: But I think the other aspect is also very important, a relationship with somebody like a teacher, not necessarily a psychiatrist that we pay, because then you might say the therapist is praising me just because I'm paying him or her, but someone who sincerely wants to help you and takes you seriously, who makes you feel you are worthy of being helped. This relational aspect is very important for Westerners, since we've been raised so much in isolation and everyone feels so lonely.

DANIEL GOLEMAN: For instance, when Western students find a teacher who is very loving and very accepting, that's very healing for this problem of low self-esteem, because they feel loved for themselves, as they are, and that helps them get over this feeling.

DALAI LAMA: So possibly a major cause of this low self-esteem is simply lack of being loved.

DANIEL BROWN: Yes, and being loved in the right way. With conditional love, where the child is loved only if he or she does the right things, the child learns that he or she is valued and respected only if the child behaves in a certain way.

JON KABAT-ZINN: And that way is the way some parents want it to be.

ALEX BERZIN: There's another important factor in Western child-raising. Children are rewarded for being bad. If you cry enough and you act in a horrible way, then your parents will finally give in and give you what you want.

DALAI LAMA: That may be much more widespread. The Tibetans seem to do that as well. [*laughter*]

FRANCISCO VARELA: Don't you find, Your Holiness, that is also true among Tibetan families, that love is perhaps not always unconditional? That parents also have their own obscurations, and therefore they're not completely able to love their children unconditionally?

DALAI LAMA: Generally, the Tibetan attitude is that parents' love toward their children is not so much based on the feeling that "My child is good," but rather, "This is my child." I think that's the main reason. This love is based on the fact that the child is one's own, and the love simply increases if the child improves and cultivates good qualities. If the child has bad qualities, and continues with those, then the love may diminish. Perhaps there could be some sociological factors. For instance, the capitalist economic system of the West is very competitive, and many of its values are considered in terms of economic consequences, so that pattern may be extended to the parent-child relationship. In the economic system, you give some money and you get something in return, and that may even be applied to children's behavior. It's almost like a business transaction: For children to receive their parents' compassion, the children should pay something, such as respect, or a nice attitude.

LEE YEARLEY: I would like to offer a different view on this, with which my colleagues may not agree. I do think that there is a deep problem with self-esteem for a part of the American population. But there is another very large part of that population, who have very strong self-esteem, and who aren't simply grandiose or somehow sick. Many of them hold power. They run the country, and they do so with a forcefulness that represents a very strong sense of self, even if it's a

largely deluded one. A significant part of that country consists of people who would be better off if they had more
problems with self-esteem!

DANIEL BROWN: If you look at depression, the statistics are significant. Fifteen percent or so of the entire population are diagnosed as depressed at some point in their lives,
and depression is usually associated with low self-esteem.
That's only the people who come to clinical attention, so I
would estimate that at least a quarter of the country should
be included, at a minimum.

LEE YEARLEY: I don't question that, but I think for
another half or at least a third of the population, this is not
applicable at all; and many of those people are the ones that
make the major decisions about what the country is and
where it goes.

DALAI LAMA: Have you found any differences in this
regard in a socialist system as opposed to a capitalist system?

DANIEL BROWN: We don't know. But there have been
some family studies concerning low self-esteem. One pattern
that emerges in a number of studies is that families with very
high expectations, particularly those that are upwardly mo-
bile, are likely to raise children with problems of low self-
esteem. Of course, after the economic depression in the
1930s, Americans were anxious that their children would not
suffer the way they had, and would achieve economic stability. Each child has his or her own temperament, his or her
own way of growing and developing. Much like the body,
there's a certain identity that's unique to an individual. In
families where there are very high expectations that a child
should grow up to be a certain way, there's a discrepancy.
Parents keep misperceiving the child and imposing expectations different from the way the child would naturally develop. The outcome is that the child, while growing up, feels
missed or not perceived correctly, as if they're not known for
who they are. This results in this self-doubt and the failure to

perceive their own value and worth. It's only one example, but it's been thoroughly studied in America.

ALEX BERZIN: From my experience in socialist countries, I find it's not so much the economic system that makes the difference. Each country seems to have its own culture. Polish people really don't care what anybody says, and in Russia, with the Orthodox Christian background, they don't have the Western problem of guilt. Each culture, each country is quite different.

DALAI LAMA: So, in answer to your initial question about beginning the cultivation of loving kindness directed toward oneself, and whether this has a place in Buddhist practice: Yes, it does. [*laughter*]

NOTES

1. *Shravaka* means hearer. These are Buddhist practitioners who practice a path of individual liberation, without the Bodhisattva resolve to become enlightened for the benefit of all beings.

2. *Pratyekabuddha* means silent buddha. These are Buddhist practitioners who have pursued a path of solitary realization. In their outlook, pratyekabuddhas understand the sense in which personality and mental events are fluid and impersonal, not rooted in a fixed self.

The Nature of Awareness

10

Mind, Brain, and Body
in Dialogue

ONE CENTRAL ISSUE is the relationship between
emotions, cognition, and brain activity, which leads to the
question of the nature of awareness or consciousness. This
is a key point on which science and Buddhism diverge:
whether consciousness is an emergent property of the
brain, or has a separate existence in its most subtle form.

The central disagreement between Buddhism and Western neuroscience revolves around the nature of consciousness. In the West, neuroscientists believe the problem of
explaining consciousness can be solved by identifying neural correlates of consciousness in the brain. One prominent
theory holds this can be accomplished by locating circuits
of neurons associated with aspects of consciousness and
determining how they are interconnected with other circuits. This model assumes consciousness emerges from the
vast interplay of countless neural networks of cells.

Still, neuroscientists acknowledge that at the present
time no one knows how a complex assembly of neurons
can be aware of itself. And some critics observe that neuro-   ←
science research assumes reductionism—the view that

mental events and behavior can be reduced to physiology. There is a healthy and active debate in contemporary science concerning the "hard problem" of consciousness, that which seems to escape explanation in terms of physiological processes. There is no agreed upon solution today.

By contrast, one Tibetan Buddhist model proposes eight varieties of consciousness: the consciousness of the "universal ground" (*Kun shi*), thought (*sems*), and the six senses. The basic duality of subjectivity, the perception of self distinct from objects of awareness, emerges at the level of the universal ground. *Sems* is cognition, the core of discursive thoughts. As the "sixth sense," cognition acts to coordinate and synthesize the other five-sense consciousnesses.

In Buddhism, meditation is used to stabilize and examine the mind carefully, finally coming to recognize subtle aspects of mind beyond the sense perceptions and thought. The dominant Western belief that consciousness is an emergent function of brain activity is a reductionist, materialist position from the Buddhist perspective. Buddhism asserts that although many forms of consciousness are associated with the brain and sensory perception, some subtle elements of consciousness are not limited to brain activity. An "intrinsic awareness" is beyond ordinary consciousness; the "Buddha nature" of all beings, it is not dependent on the body or the brain. These two positions are background to the intellectual tension in the conversation begun by a pointed inquiry by the Dalai Lama.

DALAI LAMA: Could it be possible that certain mental activities or conceptualizations themselves act as causes to stimulate parts of the brain? In other words, can there be two-way traffic? If we take as a hypothesis that consciousness does exist, there is a possibility of explaining the physiological factors. I think there are different levels of consciousness or mind. One is a product of the physical body, and that particular mind only develops in response to changes in the body. Another more subtle level of mind precedes the body and causes changes to take place in the brain. If we assume that consciousness does not exist as a separate phenomenon, but only as an emergent property of the brain, then what is the causal agent for the brain activity?

FRANCISCO VARELA: There is not an agreed-upon answer, but the general feeling in neuroscience is that consciousness is an emergent property of the intrinsic electrical activity of the brain. The idea of a more subtle mind would not be considered either necessary or provable.

DALAI LAMA: What would be the causal agent for the emergence? Are you simply saying that activation in the brain acts on other activation in the brain?

FRANCISCO VARELA: Yes. That makes a lot of sense from a scientific point of view, because you have things that impinge on each other from the very beginning. With nourishment, the brain keeps this mutual activation going.

DALAI LAMA: So, the emotions emerge because of the activity that takes place in the brain. But there is a crucial point here. Is it a causal relationship or simply a correspondence? Does the brain activity cause the emotion, or are they in fact simultaneous, without one being caused by the other?

CLIFF SARON: I wouldn't say they're simultaneous, particularly if you look at the neuroanatomy.

DALAI LAMA: Is it unequivocally and invariably the case that the brain activity precedes the emotional states?

CLIFF SARON: Brain activity exists at many different levels, and the activity at different levels causes the emotional states. Whether the differences in the cortex precede or follow the experience is a question to pursue. We can look specifically at the activity just before the facial expression and see whether it tends to correspond. In the experiments on depression and temperament, the brain differences were not related to current emotional responses, but rather to tendencies of emotional response. In that case, we can't say that the brain activity is causative for the current emotional state.

DALAI LAMA: Isn't it the case that when you go down to the most elementary level, to elementary particles, for example, that the elementary particles one finds in the human brain are indistinguishable from the elementary particles you find in stone?

FRANCISCO VARELA: The same, up to atoms and molecules.

DALAI LAMA: As you move from the elementary-particle level up through atoms, molecules, and so forth, at what level do you start speaking of the emergence of awareness?

FRANCISCO VARELA: Your Holiness, there is no consensus in neuroscience even as to what awareness is.

DALAI LAMA: Coming from the level of elementary particles on up, at what point do you find evidence for the presence of awareness?

FRANCISCO VARELA: This is something people have done research on. Evidently, everybody accepts that humans have awareness.

DALAI LAMA: When many particles join together, they become lifelike, don't they? There are two categories, plants and animals, and both have life. But one category of organisms developed awareness, and the other did not. What's the main cause for this, and at what stage does it occur?

FRANCISCO VARELA: The classical answer, and I think a very good answer, is that cognition or awareness (whatever it may be) is an emergent property of a specific pattern, or aggregation, or systemic configuration, which requires a nervous system. It requires sensory and motor devices and interneurons. Plants never developed nervous systems, but animals did. The nervous system then evolved and created different capacities for cognition. At one point, something happened—that's the big debate—that made humans aware. Most people would agree there is awareness and also compassion in some animals, such as the great apes or dolphins.

DALAI LAMA: I feel your usage of the term *awareness* is a bit too lofty, because we all certainly agree that a lot of other animals are conscious in some sense of the term, maybe even going down to the hydra.

FRANCISCO VARELA: Yes, but you cannot say they are conscious of themselves.

DALAI LAMA: I'm not referring to consciousness of themselves, but rather awareness in any sense of the term. Animals are sentient beings in that they feel, they experience.

FRANCISCO VARELA: I'm sorry. Whenever you use the word *aware* in the neuroscientific context, it has the connotation of self-awareness. You could use the term cognition or perception and everyone would agree that animals with nervous systems have a form of cognition. Many people would even say that unicellular animals like the ameba have a very primitive form of cognition.

DALAI LAMA: But plants don't?

FRANCISCO VARELA: No. The main difference, Your Holiness, has to do with a sensorimotor correlation, so there must be some possibility of motion. In behavior, this is a key element that allows us to recognize cognition. Since amoebas can move around and search for their food, they are very different from a plant that receives it passively. Being able to move around creates the possibility of a nervous system. Beyond that, it's difficult to say where it begins or ends. For example, the sum of the B- and T-cells could be said to have a very minor form of cognition, knowledge, and also stimulation.

DALAI LAMA: So, when you were saying some scientists agree great apes also had awareness, you meant self-awareness similar to humans.

FRANCISCO VARELA: Yes, a form of self-reflection that might be similar to our own experience. This probably would not be the case for a cat, or less so, and even less for an ameba.

Emotions Triggered by Thoughts

Cliff Saron: Your Holiness, we've talked about internal causes and external causes of emotion, but what movement of mind specifically triggers an emotion?

Dalai Lama: It is difficult to say. One can ask first of all whether emotions exist in the mind of an *arhat,* a liberated being, or in a buddha who is free of all obscurations. If one includes things like loving kindness and compassion as emotions, then the answer has to be yes, those are present in the mind of a highly enlightened being. So you can't say, for example, that egotism is a necessary cause in the arising of emotions, because enlightened beings don't have egotism, but they do have emotion. A sense of self is not necessarily deluded, as egotism is, so enlightened beings may have a nondeluded sense of self. But it's an open question whether that triggers emotion, or whether emotion is simply in the nature of awareness itself, or whether it's triggered by the apprehension of a specific object.

There are different levels of consciousness. On the one hand, there is a level of consciousness that is very directly contingent on the body. For example, there are cases in which a physical dysfunction, such as an imbalance in the body, is the chief cause for mental distortion such as craving.

Now, if you look at sensory perception, Buddhist psychology speaks of three types of contributing causes, which together give rise to the continuum of sensory awareness. For example, in visual perception, the first cause, known as the dominant condition, is the physical visual faculty. Second, there's the referential condition, which is the external stimulus. The third cause, called the immediate condition, is the immediately preceding event of clarity or the knowing quality in the sensory perception. This event of clarity also has its contributing causes, and its immediate cause is the preceding moment of perception. So, one of the three conditions is cognitive, this preceding moment of perception.

From experience, it's certainly true that you can be sitting very quietly with no particular stimulus coming in, when a thought arises and causes you to be startled or jump, or have some kind of physical reaction. It seems that first of all there is a subjective cognitive event, which then acts as the cause for the physical, and not vice versa. Then, of course, it can also happen that activity within the body enhances that emotion, and it can also modify or change the emotion. It is common experience that awareness seems, by its nature, to be vacillating or fluctuating. It seems to be oscillating even faster than ten cycles per second. [*laughter*] Now, in meditation, the cultivation of mindfulness serves to contain one's awareness and dampens the vacillations so the awareness or attention can become stable. If this is the case, it would seem that the very nature of awareness has been changed by freshly introducing this purely subjective mental means, namely the cultivation of mindfulness. It seems plausible that this in itself would also bring about changes in the brain and in the body as a whole.

FRANCISCO VARELA: In that case, does the emotional state cause the vacillation in awareness?

DALAI LAMA: In terms of causal sequence, you first of all have the basic contact, then you have the actual cognition, and this induces the emotion.

FRANCISCO VARELA: So the emotion comes after the ascertainment. What about the situation when, for example, we suddenly hear a sound, a crack, and the attention changes? It seems we first have some kind of alert, panic, fear—an emotional state—and only after that, we realize that the roof is about to fall. Doesn't the emotion precede the ascertainment in this case?

DALAI LAMA: If you did a very precise momentary analysis, it seems you would find some cognition of something happening there. You hear an anomalous sound, even if you haven't identified it as the roof collapsing, and this incites the emotion. Then comes the more detailed awareness of what's going on. It's a matter of complexity: you do apprehend the sound, but only later do you know what it might mean.

FRANCISCO VARELA: How would you analyze the situation at the other extreme, when there is no particular event? You are just sitting there, or walking, when a change of mood occurs. All of a sudden you feel lonely, or maybe depressed, or happy, or whatever. What would be the contributing cause for that emotion shift?

DALAI LAMA: It may be thoroughly internal, or it may be very subtly externally induced. On the one hand, we have accustomed ourselves to certain habits of conceptualization that build up predilections. So, even in the absence of any explicit external stimuli, the force of your previous habituation may give rise to a seemingly spontaneous shift of mood. Another possibility is that the environment may have some very subtle quality that arouses this emotion. It could be subtly pleasant or have some kind of faintly depressing quality to it, even though you may not consciously be aware of it.

On my first visit to Moscow, my mental function was very dull. Other Tibetan lamas who visited that area have described a similar experience of unprecedented emotion during their daily prayers. Of course, it might have been because breakfast was very late that morning. [*laughter*] But unfortunately in that area, there has been so much killing, so much negative human emotion. In that situation, even though there's nothing manifest or evident that you're conscious of, the effect can still be there. You can translate it roughly as gloom, but literally it means something that obscures, or veils, or clouds [Tib.: *sgrib pa*]. Likewise, Tibetan practitioners who remain in the mountains can usually predict when somebody is about to come, either the next day or later in the evening. This definitely happens, so there's some influence from the environment, whether negative or positive, even though it's not a conscious stimulus.

DANIEL BROWN: Some Western theories of emotion also talk about different levels of information processing.

They may not agree on whether the cognition takes place on a preattentive level, before it is conscious, or after conscious recognition when the thought is more elaborated. But there's a common assumption, as in the Tibetan tradition, that there is always some cognition involved.

DANIEL GOLEMAN: A study done by Richard Davidson throws some light on repression and brain function. You know that the right side of the body is controlled by the left side of the brain, and vice versa. That's true also for what you see, so if you divide what comes into each eye into a left side and right side, what comes into the right side goes to the left side of the brain and what comes into the left side goes to the right side of the brain. In this study, they used a device to show a word to one side of the brain or the other side. Words shown to the right side go into the left side of the brain, where the center that controls speech is located. On the right side of the brain, as Cliff told us, is the center for negative emotion. This means that if the word you see on the right side is upsetting to you, the information about what that word is goes first to the left side of the brain and then to the right, where the emotional reaction occurs. They were able to measure the exact time lag between activity on the left and right sides, and a very interesting thing happened. With a neutral word like *glass* there was no difference between the repressors and the other people. With a very disturbing word such as *kill* there was a noticeable increase for repressors in the time that information took to get across from one side to the other. This may mean that somewhere in the brain there's something like a censor that says, "You can't print that; you can't know that." So it may be true that repressors actually do not experience what they are denying.

DALAI LAMA: What happens if you show that same word to the left side of the eye?

CLIFF SARON: It would project from the left visual field to the right side of the brain. These were right-handed people whose speech apparatus is presumably controlled by regions of the left side of the brain, so in order for them to speak, the information would have to transfer from the right side to the left side.

DALAI LAMA: How about a pleasant word? Is that the same as a neutral word in terms of the speed with which it goes from right to left?

DANIEL GOLEMAN: I don't believe there were differences between pleasant words and neutral words. The finding of the study was that neutral words, when presented directly to the left side of the brain, produced a certain speed of response that was not different from that of pleasant words, but unpleasant words presented to the right side of the brain were slower than pleasant words.

CLIFF SARON: The idea was that this censor decreased the transfer of negative emotional information from the right to the left side of the brain, where we are allowed to speak the response.

DANIEL GOLEMAN: I don't know if we can say where the censor is located, if anywhere.

CLIFF SARON: The test was a free-association test: you see a word and you have to say the first word that comes to your mind. The measurement that we're taking is not an electrical measurement of the brain but of how long it takes to speak. It's the reaction time.

DALAI LAMA: For instance, if a neutral word is shown on your left, it goes to the right side.

CLIFF SARON: That's right. It will always take a little longer for a word that goes to the left visual field to be spoken.

FRANCISCO VARELA: If there is always a reaction time, why should one speak of censorship? Strictly speaking, it would be more like a sluggishness than a censorship.

CLIFF SARON: There's a gate. It takes time to go over, or to lift it up.

DANIEL GOLEMAN: You could say there's just more processing going on for unpleasant words than for pleasant words. We don't exactly know more than that.

BOB LIVINGSTON: His Holiness may be interested to know that all of us have some degree of censorship operating on seeing words and pictures, and I'll give two examples. A combination of words like *hero* and *fame* are seen very quickly, with a short reaction time. A combination like *lady* and *slut* takes about four times as long to read in milliseconds. This is true for all of us in a normal population. If you ask a person to identify what he or she sees in a picture, it makes a great difference whether it's a pleasant picture or one that gives rise to negative feelings. If you show four pictures in a group and ask people to tell you as soon as they can identify any of them, they see the positive pictures very quickly. But it may take a whole second to be able to see a negative picture. This is an operation that occurs before awareness.

DANIEL GOLEMAN: Since you're interested, I'll tell you about another study. When you focus or look at something, the eye makes tiny little movements. Ophthalmologists have a device that allows them to track the eye's movements exactly, without interfering with what you see. When people who were known to be very anxious looked at a picture that had both unpleasant and neutral sections, the eye would go only to the neutral area. It wouldn't even look at the unpleasant area. When asked what was in the picture, they would describe all the pleasant things, but have no memory of the unpleasant things. We don't know exactly how that happens, but it suggests again that prior to full awareness, part of the brain can know what's going on and guide perception away from something unpleasant.

DALAI LAMA: From a Buddhist point of view, the question would be whether the person hasn't seen that image or cannot recall it. It might be that the person has visually seen it, but because he or she hasn't paid enough attention to that particular section, the person hasn't made the connection. So, at the sensory level, there is no judgment involved.

DANIEL GOLEMAN: This is the point. Sometimes it's true that the person doesn't see it at all. That's what they could tell with this device. Other times they may see it, but they don't recall it.

DALAI LAMA: How can you tell the difference?

JON KABAT-ZINN: In point of fact, the experiment is showing you that they do see it. If the eye-tracking movements did not censor, they would distribute over the whole field. In this case, you're finding that these people's eyes are selecting for the pleasant, which tells you they have to have seen it.

DANIEL GOLEMAN: That's the next point.

CLIFF SARON: There is a point of clarification I could make, Your Holiness. The device that's used tracks the center of vision, the very small area of the clearest vision. But you also see information with your peripheral vision, which informs you very consciously not to move in that direction.

SENSORY PERCEPTION AND CONSCIOUSNESS

FRANCISCO VARELA: It's also fair to say there is an enormous amount of judgment made at what we call very low-level vision, even at the level of the eye or just the retina. For example, already in the retina you can determine where there is an edge and where there is none, before it's a fully configured object, for example. You won't know whether it is a glass or a microphone, but if there is an edge in your visual field, that is already an important decision made in a few milliseconds. That's very important from the neuroscientific point of view. The building-up of the full visual field happens at many stages. What is low can be very elaborate, with a lot of judgment, construction, and interpretation involved, even way before awareness. — *memory is constantly automatic.*

DALAI LAMA: Before the information even reaches the brain?

FRANCISCO VARELA: The image that goes out from the optic nerve is not the raw set of light that has come onto the retina. It's already extremely textured and elaborated before it reaches the central brain.

DALAI LAMA: But isn't the position of modern neuroscience that it's not actually the eye but the brain that sees?

FRANCISCO VARELA: It is neither the brain nor the eye, but the fact that the two of them are working together. As much as there is activity going up from the eye to the brain, there is activity going down from brain out toward the senses. There is as much of what we call the central control of sensory afference as there is of the sensory afference that goes into the brain. It is the coming together of these two things that makes vision, so it is neither in the eye nor in the brain. It's everywhere; it's an emerging property.

DALAI LAMA: The question is whether there is a possibility of judgment within visual perception, independent of mental perception. There seems to be some uncertainty as to whether this is asserted in the Prasangika system, which we regard as the most sophisticated philosophical system in Buddhism. What is certain, from the Prasangika perspective, is that the appearances to the various senses are already tainted by the influence or latent propensity of one's previous ignorance, grasping onto existence as true. Appearances certainly do affect the various senses, and these senses are not mental awareness. But it remains an open question whether, in terms of their actual mode of apprehending objects, the various senses are in any way modified by judgment.

FRANCISCO VARELA: The neuroscientific point of view would say, absolutely, that they are. When you touch your skin, for example, the activity of the receptor that feels is under direct control of the upper brain. The brain regulates what constitutes data. For a neuroscientist, what counts as information coming from the senses is always a two-way affair: both the impact of my finger, and the control of the receptor that interprets the impact. Even at that low level, beyond the point of sensory impact, there is an enormous amount of treatment of this activity.[1] For example, in the retina, what goes out from the optic nerve is not just the activity of the receptor. If we could compare images of receptor activity and nerve activity, the two would look very different. Edges and demarcations of textures and surfaces would already appear at this level.

ALAN WALLACE: Are you saying that even very primitive visual awareness is conditioned by previous experience?

FRANCISCO VARELA: Some low-level treatment is not even dependent on previous experience, it's just wired in.

CLIFF SARON: It's a function of the way the cells are connected.

FRANCISCO VARELA: For example, when you look at the optic nerve in the retina of a frog, you see activity that pertains only to things that count as flies. You don't see these "fly detectors" in the retina of humans or monkeys.

DALAI LAMA: If, for example, you're suddenly burned, and the limb naturally contracts very rapidly, and pulls away from the source of heat, is this immediate reaction connected to the brain or is it not?

FRANCISCO VARELA: Both are true. If the connection to the brain is cut and your leg is burned, it will still contract, because that's a low-level reflex. It is also true that the low-level reflex is normally under modulation of the higher centers, so that if you are burned, the low-level reflex overrides the higher control. Afterward, the higher control can say, "You're exaggerating, it wasn't that bad." There are levels of interdependence, and different levels are more important at different points on a continuum. Immediately on burning, the low-level reflex takes over; the higher centers take over in normal activity such as walking. At the opposite extreme of the continuum is the artist walking on a tightrope in a circus, who performs a creative act in using higher levels to resist the very strong tendencies of the low-level reflexes.

Whatever counts as a perception is not really localized, but is in fact a collective affair with everybody doing their part. That's very important in neuroscience. By and large, the brain works as a distributive device. We speak about localization only because when you damage a location, you stop a function, and not because it works right there and only there. It's a common mistake; the language we use to describe this reduces it to something that isn't true.

NOTES

1. In the example of the visual system, the receptors are the rods and cones of the retina. Rods cannot detect color, but are sensitive to light intensity. Cones detect color and mediate detailed and accurate vision. There are four different types of nerves in the retina, which are functionally distinct. These send information to the optic nerve, which sends it to the visual cortex via the thalamic nucleus. Sensor and receptor are synonymous in this context.

11

Subtleties of Consciousness

IN THE TERMINOLOGY of philosopher of science Thomas Kuhn, Buddhism and neuroscience represent differing *paradigms:* bodies of laws, methods, and theories within a discipline that generate a coherent intellectual outlook. Just as neuroscientists are trained within a paradigm that has its characteristic methods and theories, Buddhist scholars and practitioners are trained in a very different body of theory and utilize methods like meditation to explore a territory also covered by neuroscience: the landscape of consciousness.

The Dalai Lama discusses phenomena such as after-death experiences and meditative states that could challenge the paradigm of Western neuroscience by pointing to subtleties of consciousness unknown to neuroscience. Normal science involves puzzle-solving within a dominant paradigm. Periodically, new discoveries do not fit the paradigm; as a result, the old paradigm must be discarded and a new paradigm must replace it. The Dalai Lama—while acknowledging the possibility that scientific data from the West could shift the Buddhist paradigm—hints that there are phenomena beyond the frontier of science which could result in such a paradigm shift for Western science. (Some of these issues are evoked in this discussion, and they were systematically explored at the following Mind and Life Conference, "Sleeping, Dreaming, and Dying.")

DALAI LAMA: If scientific research results in empirical evidence that directly controverts some statement that one finds in the Buddhist Sutras, it would be unreasonable to hold tenaciously to the Buddhist views. However, the mere absence of empirical scientific confirmation is no reason to throw out the Buddhist assertions. Rather, you need something that directly, empirically controverts the Buddhist position before you are compelled to dismiss that position. The traditional Mahayana approach toward its own tenets would be to examine them critically—be they assertions about cosmology or whatever—compare them to scientific evidence, and see whether the Buddhist assertions can be taken literally or whether they must be freshly interpreted. As soon as you say that the Buddha's teachings fall into two categories—those that are to be taken literally, and those that must be interpreted to find the true meaning—you must then place the chief priority on reason and not rely simply on the authority of the scriptures.

FRANCISCO VARELA: Of course, whether there is empirical evidence that contradicts the points of the tradition is very difficult to evaluate. It is hard to say what will be counted as evidence and when it will be accepted. For example, for some scientists, it is a fact that there is no mind beyond the brain. What counts as evidence for the Buddhists doesn't count as a fact for some scientists. Both sides will say they have evidence, and of course they're seeing different worlds. The inner ear and the sense of balance, which counts as a sense in the West but not in classical Buddhism is perhaps a simple example, but then more difficult examples are where the interpretation would have to come in.

DALAI LAMA: That's a fundamental issue right there, the mind and the mind-brain relationship. My perspective on

this is that there are many degrees of subtlety of consciousness, and science has looked only at the ordinary levels. So,
science has merely not found the more subtle ones, which are
crucial to the Buddhist presentations, and merely not finding
is not enough to controvert. As I think I mentioned earlier,
because of the human body, there is a certain consciousness
that entirely depends on the human organism. Obviously, we
call that grosser level of mind the human mind. In that sense,
you could virtually speak of the human mind as being an
emergent property of the body. But now how did the human
mind become a mind? You would have to say, in general, a
continuity of awareness does exist.

FRANCISCO VARELA: That's precisely the inference
that most Western neuroscientists would not be willing to
make. They would interpret that inference as based on ideo-
logical or religious belief and discount it as nonevidence.
They would ask what your evidence is for the existence of
awareness.

DALAI LAMA: The Buddhist position here is not utterly without evidence. For example, first of all, there are
those who recall their former lives; secondly, there are those
who have heightened awareness, or clairvoyance; and thirdly,
there are people who have utterly extraordinary qualities,
even from infancy. All these can be counted as evidence. Concerning the whole universe, with one galaxy disappearing and
another galaxy developing, we can ask about the causes of
these phenomena. Scientists, of course, have their Big Bang
theory. Nevertheless, I think there are still a lot of mysterious
phenomena remaining to be explained. Then, either you accept that the first things in the universe came without cause,
which is not a satisfactory answer; or if you accept God, this
still remains controversial from the Buddhist viewpoint. Of
course, the Buddhist explanation is also not completely satisfactory—a lot of questions remain. In science, phenomena
are explained according to a paradigm that does not accept
the existence of mind independent of the brain. But it's an
open question whether all these types of extraordinary experiences can be explained within that paradigm.

FRANCISCO VARELA: Yes, except that, as you know, every bit of evidence can be reconceptualized. For example, people who recall former lives in the West would normally be taken to a psychiatric clinic and treated as delusional schizophrenics. Nobody would pay attention to that because it's simply craziness. Some schizophrenics have discourse that perhaps when looked at from the point of view of Buddhist or other mystical traditions seems the discourse of a very enlightened person. So you see, somebody's evidence is somebody else's disease.

DALAI LAMA: I think there are two levels of truth. One type of truth becomes public consensus. But there's another sort of truth that is not established by consensus. Certainly, there can be truths right now that no one in the world knows about. They are still truths, aren't they? It's not necessary that someone accept them as truth. Within that same context, there can be some truths that only a very few people have realized, because they have known something directly for themselves. It doesn't need to be known by everyone in order to be true. Concerning your point about certain unusual experiences counting as evidence in one discipline, while counting as error in another, this is where research is extremely important.

PARADIGMS AND THE "FACTS" THEY REVEAL

FRANCISCO VARELA: The kind of truth that science adheres to is a very limited model of truth. This is truth by consensus taken to its extreme. The beauty of science is that it builds this truth by consensus very effectively, through experiments, in publications, in conferences and such. Its weakness is that it has no place for the other kind of truth.

DALAI LAMA: Perhaps it's also possible to understand that scientific inquiry and other types of inquiry, such as religious inquiry, are operating within quite different fields of reference. For instance, scientific inquiry is mainly done within the framework of taking measurements of physical phenomena. And even within science, you have two categories, hard science and soft science. For example, if you were to make [some of the clinical] presentations you gave here within the context of hard science, what would be the response?

JON KABAT-ZINN: Not too good! [*laughter*]

DANIEL BROWN: Yes, but even with hard science, Your Holiness, there are limitations. Once I was doing some research on meditators and an accomplished meditator from another Buddhist tradition posed a very interesting question to me: "Do you have a machine that can measure awareness?" I think as long as we don't have technology that can measure awareness, we probably won't understand the mind with science. That doesn't mean it's not a truth or it doesn't exist, it means that we don't have the technology, and hard science needs to appreciate that limitation.

DALAI LAMA: So, until we can actually ascertain the nature of awareness, it's difficult, and that itself is the hard question.

DANIEL GOLEMAN: I wonder if this subtle consciousness you mentioned is beyond the reach of science. You have here a group of eager scientists who would be interested in hearing a little more about subtle consciousness as you mean it, to see if it might be studied. Perhaps we could use the methods of hard science to establish your case in this argument about whether mind exists.

DALAI LAMA: I personally have nothing to say, as I can't speak from profound meditative experience. But based on the Buddhist treatises, I can say that the issue of subtle consciousness is related to two potential fields of research. One is research on people in the dream state, and the other is on people in the dying process. Two other pertinent types of experience worthy of research are deep sleep when one is not dreaming, and the experience of fainting.

SUBTLETIES OF CONSCIOUSNESS:
THE TIBETAN VIEW

ADAM ENGLE: The interesting point is that if you investigate the body by using the mind in meditation, you come upon the energy system first before you reach the cellular and chemical levels. However, if you investigate with microscopes and other instruments, you come upon the cellular and chemical levels first. This may explain why Eastern systems have described the channels[1] only, and Western science has described the cellular and chemical levels.

DANIEL BROWN: What do the meditators who are very skilled at both perceiving and transforming energy currents have to say about the cellular system? Does their perception of bodily changes eventually extend to the cellular changes [in the immune system] that Francisco described?

DALAI LAMA: There's no question that skilled yogis or contemplatives can perceive the various energies in the body, including the five principal and five secondary energies, and even the colors associated with those energies. So in principle it is possible for them also to use their *samadhi*[2] to perceive the cellular level.

DANIEL BROWN: Can they also ascertain chemical changes?

DALAI LAMA: The *bindhu,* or drops[3], within the body are another issue. These tend to have the connotation of substance rather than energy, and these also are identified in the yogic practice.

FRANCISCO VARELA: If the yogi can identify activity on the cellular level, then by implication he or she should also be able to follow the cellular activity in the brain. In that case, we would have a fantastic "cerebroscope."

DALAI LAMA: One can easily ask why the Buddhist contemplative scriptures do not include an elaborate description of the brain functions and cellular functions. One possible reason is that the chief emphasis is on understanding the mind, and what is instrumental or essential to that. This includes the chakras—the channels[4]—and the drops, and it stops there.

DANIEL GOLEMAN: I'm intrigued by your statement that the yogi would know this through *samadhi.* What is the mechanism or organ of knowing? How could the yogi know the brain in intimate detail unless the brain itself was the basis for that knowing?

DALAI LAMA: The Buddhist presentation speaks of the brain as the basis for awareness, but the brain doesn't really know anything at all. The awareness knows things, and one of those things might be the cellular level of the body.

ROBERT THURMAN: Might the awareness that perceives the physical structure of one's own brain be the subtlest level of consciousness?

HEIGHTENED SENSORY AWARENESS AS A RESULT OF MEDITATIVE PRACTICE

DALAI LAMA: Even at a grosser level, at a point in tantric realization known as isolation of the speech, where the practitioner still hasn't experienced the most subtle clear-light state of mind—even at that point it's possible to perceive the energies directly, and their associated colors.

DANIEL GOLEMAN: But isn't that perception independent of the usual modes of perception such as the visual system?

DALAI LAMA: It's mental.

DANIEL GOLEMAN: Purely mental without involving the brain at all?

DALAI LAMA: It's an interesting issue. On the one hand, as I said previously, the brain might act as the dominant condition for these various types of mental awareness arising, just as the visual mechanism is the dominant condition for the perception. But it also occurred to me that the *Kalachakra-tantra* speaks of a new sensory or cognitive faculty that arises freshly in the course of contemplative development. Whether that is material or immaterial, we don't know.

So there are two different interpretations, depending on whether the context is Sutra or Vajrayana.[5] In the Sutra context, the various types of heightened awareness arise by the power of *samadhi*. They are purely of a cognitive nature, arising from the mind, and this interpretation speaks only of heightened visual or auditory awareness. Olfactory, gustatory, and tactile sensations are different in that the sensory organ has to contact its object. In the Vajrayana, or Tantra, context it's said that various types of heightened awareness can be induced by the power of *prana*, or energy.[6] These are physical causes, not just cognitive. In a tantric system of meditation that exploits or manipulates the subtle energies and the energy channels, it is possible to cultivate heightened awareness for all five senses, not just the visual and auditory.

DANIEL GOLEMAN: If you had a yogi who was doing this, and you measured his brain, would there be specific brain changes related to this?

DALAI LAMA: Yes. You get the equipment ready, and we'll bring the yogis.

DANIEL GOLEMAN: It's a deal.

DANIEL BROWN: To summarize, Tibetan Buddhism takes a pragmatic point of view, in the same sense that Lee Yearley described William James's pragmatism: the point of any study is what's useful or of benefit. It's conceivable that a skilled yogi could perceive the brain and chemical activity, but this activity is not the most important thing to study from the perspective of the goal, which is enlightenment for all sentient beings. Is it fair to say that this is why such study has not been emphasized?

DALAI LAMA: Even though it might not have been important in the past, it is now. [*laughter*]

ROBERT THURMAN: If we hypothesize that the experience of yogis in the past, including the Buddha, who was the best yogi of all, informs the Buddhist tradition of medicine, then it may have been by choice rather than ignorance that the cellular level was not used in the same way as in Western medicine. The fruitful question, then, is why they chose not to intervene at the molecular level or the cellular level except with herbal medicine, and worked mostly at the energetic level. There may be a lesson there.

DALAI LAMA: We might have to travel back in time and ask that question of the Buddha himself! But it could be that the cellular level is superficial, and instead they wanted to go down to something deeper.

FRANCISCO VARELA: It's not obvious why the yogi should encounter the energy level first rather than the cellular level, which is the most immediate from the Western point of view.

DALAI LAMA: One reason could be that *lung*, or energy as defined in the Buddhist tantric literature, is the mount or the vehicle through which consciousness and mental events occur. But it's also the case that you can follow this energy even to the most subtle levels of consciousness, and at that level you've really left behind the gross physical level of cellular activity.

FRANCISCO VARELA: Which would suggest that treating *lung* as energy in the same sense as electromagnetic or other energy might be what Whitehead called the fallacy of misplaced concreteness.

DALAI LAMA: By understanding and manipulating these energies, you can have a direct effect on the mental states, which is why the yogis emphasized their importance. Further, influencing your mind or changing your mental state can also affect the physiological state of your body. It doesn't work the other way around. A change in physiological state does not necessarily affect your mind, especially at the subtlest levels. But the reality of the situation is that we don't know whether the yogis perceive the cellular level, and if so why they don't talk about it.

SUBTLE ENERGY IN LIFE AND DEATH

JON KABAT-ZINN: Your Holiness, you asked a very interesting question earlier that I think surprised all the Westerners: What happens to the nervous system and the immune system when a person dies? We are now talking about a third system, which is really modeled on solid state physics. This model does not necessarily relate to the living properties of a structure, but is of a different order of magnitude. Given that there's a direct connection between the experience of meditators and practitioners of Tibetan medicine, I would like to ask now whether you have any sense of what happens to the subtle energy system at death?

DALAI LAMA: You'll find slightly different presentations in various Tantras, depending perhaps on different persons' metabolisms or predilections. In the death process, one speaks of the dissolution of four elements: first the earth element, corresponding to solidity; then water; fire or heat; and finally air. One's perceptual experience is the first thing to go—visual experience doesn't entirely vanish, but it becomes somewhat vague or fuzzy. In terms of external signs, the skin of the body becomes a little bit tight. I expect that the immune system and brain shut down upon the dissolution of the air element, because at that point breathing stops, and presumably very shortly afterward, the brain doesn't receive sufficient oxygen, and it dies. But after the respiration has ceased, there are still four more stages in the death process. So death does not occur simultaneously when respiration stops.

JON KABAT-ZINN: When would the subtle energy system be knocked out? From the point of view of Western physics, there's no reason why that should stop with death. The conduction system should be just as effective afterward.

DALAI LAMA: There are four further stages of the dissolution process. These are described in terms of certain visionary experiences, during which there are still some relatively subtle energies persistent. Then these gradually dissolve until finally, at the conclusion of the eighth stage, the most subtle energy is no longer present in the body. This extremely subtle energy doesn't simply vanish and become nonexistent, but rather it separates from the body. Its reliance on the body is now severed. This severing of the dependence of the subtle energy from the body is used in the Tibetan Buddhist practices on the transference of consciousness.

JON KABAT-ZINN: So if the energy system does in fact exist, it may actually be possible to study this in people after death.

DALAI LAMA: After Western "death." The phenomenon can occur even in the case of ordinary people. The body of one lady who died remained six days, I think, without decaying. We believe that when the eighth mental state occurs, they technically are dying, but not dead. It would be interesting to do research on the differences between the brain of this so-called clinically dead person and a brain that is decomposing.

DANIEL GOLEMAN: It may not be the brain that's important; it may be this other energy system that has nothing to do with the brain.

DALAI LAMA: It would be very good to have some so-phisticated equipment that could be brought to bear to this issue. The only real problem is simply waiting for one of these yogis to die.

ROBERT THURMAN: This is a new definition of am-bulance chasing!

JON KABAT-ZINN: Can we complete this line of questioning by bringing it back to the emotions and the dis-cussion that Lee Yearley led about virtue as opposed to vice? Would the experience of this extended dying process—where Western medicine would say the person is dead, while Ti-betan medicine would say they are still dying—be a function of the person's virtue in some way balanced against their neg-ative emotions?

DALAI LAMA: This ability to abide in the clear-light state occurs in two sorts of cases. One is very straightfor-ward: it arises by the power of one's yogic realization. But there is another category that has a lot of miscellaneous cir-cumstances, at least as far as we can judge by appearances. These people are not yogis, and as far as one can ascertain (I have some acquaintances among them), they didn't experi-ence the deepest form of clear light in this lifetime. Neverthe-less they were able to abide in that state for some seven or eight days. In such cases, this ability probably is related some-how to virtue, to the force of one's own previous virtuous karmic acts.

JON KABAT-ZINN: It could be an extension of our notion of health, way beyond the Western concept. The Ti-betan meditational view of human beings is even more com-plicated than that of Western science, because there are all sorts of levels of expression of being that are hardly valued or recognized in the West. Perhaps our notions of health, of wholeness or integration as a being, are reduced somewhat from what they might be if we had a more complete perspec-tive that included this clear-light tantric understanding. Do you see any value in that?

DALAI LAMA: It's certainly interesting, and it requires further research. From the Buddhist perspective, the more explanation and insight there is here, the better.

BRAIN ACTIVITY AND MEDITATIVE STATES

DALAI LAMA: Has there been any research done on [brain activity of] people who are practicing *samatha,* or meditative quiescence?

DANIEL GOLEMAN: There are not yet very good studies of brain activity during a state of one-pointed concentration. There are, however, some good studies of the effects of *vipassana* practice. In general, they find that the calming practices turn out to be very calming physiologically. The heart rate and breath rate slow down. The body's metabolism slows down.

DANIEL BROWN: From the perspective of brain activity, we don't know what happens to emotions during calming meditation practice. I have done some studies where people report verbally on their subjective sense of what happens. We devised questionnaires and looked at how people's responses to the same questions changed over time as they gained experience with meditation. One of the things that clearly changes is the skill at attention and awareness. People find that despite internal changes in their state, they can still maintain a steadiness of awareness. The other thing that became very clear was that people developed a flexibility; when they experienced some distraction, they could bring their mind back more easily. We found that emotions continued to occur. People reported the emotion with greater intensity, but let it remain in their awareness without reacting to it as much. We looked at the reactivity on two levels: on a gross level of evaluative thoughts, such as negative judgments about what was happening, and on the more subtle level of aversion and clinging. On both levels they had less reactivity, and yet the feeling was stil! very present in their awareness, often with even greater intensity. The subjects were skilled meditators from a Western perspective, but not with the level of experience that you would find represented in the Tibetan Buddhist tradition, where people meditate much more intensively over many more years. We don't know what happens to emotions in people who are very advanced in meditation.

DANIEL GOLEMAN: In another study on concentration, it was found that when people concentrated very hard the brain became quieter, with less activity.

DALAI LAMA: What about the case of people who are normally quite dull? Is it possible to do comparative research on the brain activity of people who are mentally dull and those who are very bright and have trained the mind to a very concentrated state?

CLIFF SARON: There have been some studies of brain activity in experts who are extremely proficient at a particular task, as well as novices who are not very good at a task. The experiments show that the brain uses more energy in the case of novices, and for experts the brain seems to operate more efficiently in metabolic terms, measured as the amount of glucose the brain needs. But the whole idea of activity is a very complicated issue because of the tremendous complexity of the brain and the different ways the neural tissue can function.

DANIEL GOLEMAN: But there is a general principle that the skilled brain, whether it's a meditator or chess player, uses less energy to do a better job.

NOTES

1. Channels (*tsa*) are subtle inner conduits similar to the meridians in acupuncture. *Prana* or *lung* is the energy that moves through these channels.

2. *Samadhi* is a nondistracted state of meditation free from thoughts.

3. *Bindhu* or *thigle* (drops or essence) refers to a subtle inner essence that can be perceived as spheres of light of different sizes and colors by advanced practitioners.

4. Chakras (centers) are critical energy points, corresponding to the crown of the head, the throat, the heart, the navel, and the sex organs. These centers are linked by a central channel (*tsa uma*).

5. There are two general divisions in Tibetan Buddhism, Sutra and Tantra, both with Buddhahood as their goals. Sutra is a more gradual path, using progressive practices to purify the mind; Tantra instead uses a direct perception of the enlightened state to transform ordinary mind states.

6. *Prana* or *lung* (energy) refers to a subtle inner energy connected to the breath. According to Tantra, the activity of the mind is related to this subtle inner energy.

PART SIX

A Universal Ethic

12

Medicine and Compassion

THE DALAI LAMA

How do the principles of compassion and universal responsibility fit into the fabric of contemporary culture? The Dalai Lama, in a wide-ranging exploration of compassion, human nature, and ethics, advocates a sense of universal responsibility based on the notion that all people are human beings who wish for happiness. If we recognize that all others have the same wish for happiness and wish to avoid suffering, then we can develop greater tolerance and acceptance of others. Furthermore, the Dalai Lama concludes that human cooperation is essential. Whatever the role of the individual—be it a politician, a scientist, an industrialist, a worker, or a spiritual practitioner—the most important thing is to see the interdependence of these roles and responsibilities, and the need for mutual cooperation. Although misunderstanding plays a powerful role in the course of human events, the predominant experience is one of cooperation—without it society cannot function.

The Dalai Lama proposes that compassion is intrinsic to human nature, evident in the caring attentiveness between parents and children, in a stranger stopping to help a stranded motorist, in the friendly chatter among neighbors at a local store or post office. So the Dalai Lama concludes that compassion is a natural state of human life. Still, it must be cultivated and not taken for granted. The education of children must involve ethical training, so they can grow up to contribute to society and humanity as a whole.

The Dalai Lama begins the dialogue by emphasizing his concern about the billions of people who are in search of guiding moral principles for life, but hold no strong religious beliefs.

DALAI LAMA: We talked earlier about the 5 billion people on the planet [and how only a relatively small number have a religious faith that offers them an ethical basis for living]. My main concern is to promote genuine human qualities among people, as the most effective method, without any religious agenda. Religion is a private business, isn't it? That's why, if our moral principals and ethics are tied closely to religion, it creates a lot of problems. We all agree that we, as human beings, need to accept some moral principals and ethics. The question is, how to promote these? If they are tied to religion, then to promote those principles, there's no other choice but to promote religion. Then the question becomes, which religion? And then there are a lot of complications. It's much better if religion becomes one's own business like the color of one's clothes. It's your own choice, your own business!

LEE YEARLEY: I find something so thoroughly astonishing about the emergence of consciousness and the possibility of compassion that to simply call it natural is not fully to describe what it is. This is, in part, a religious sensibility. I'm not sure if you mean by *religious* what other religions do, but it surely seems to me not natural that beings should somehow be able to help one another or be able to reflect and transcend themselves. That is part of what I mean by religious; I would hate for the word *religious* to become the sole property of those people who belonged to particular religions, because I think we would have lost something very important in our understanding of what everyone has.

CULTIVATING COMPASSION

DANIEL GOLEMAN: Your Holiness, as Jon mentioned, compassion and empathy have been left out of medical education, although they are urgently needed. Some of us are trying to redesign medical training to include compassion and empathy for other people. We're interested if you have any thoughts on methods or approaches that might be useful for this.

DALAI LAMA: In Buddhism, medicine is classified as one of the five fields of knowledge designed for caring for others, along with technology, logic, the science of sound—which includes linguistics—and inner knowledge, or spiritual practice. There is a popular saying that the efficacy of the treatment depends not so much on the physician's expertise, but rather on the physician's altruism and compassion. I have heard people say that a certain person is a great physician, that he has great knowledge and expertise, but they have doubts about his personality. Of course, patients always find some complaint, don't they?

JON KABAT-ZINN: It's the same in the West.

DALAI LAMA: Compassion and altruism are qualities that need to be naturally drawn from within one's own inner resources. They also depend a lot on environmental factors. It is definitely helpful to come up with new initiatives, as you have in this particular field. Then if other people take a similar initiative, and it becomes established, it could have greater impact. This very much calls into question the type of attitude or outlook on life that one must adopt. A most important factor would be to expose children to the values of compassion, loving kindness, altruism, and so forth from an early age. If possible, these could be introduced in the educational curriculum in schools.

JON KABAT-ZINN: I like what you say about other people taking responsibility for doing this in various other institutions. There are many people in America who have been meditating for some time, and many of them want to use meditation for right livelihood in some way. There are no models for how to do this in America. Each time it's introduced, in a school for example, it's totally new. It could be done in many ways that are not skillful, especially in terms of attitude. Would you encourage people to be creative about moving in this attitudinal direction in the places where they work?

DALAI LAMA: You don't necessarily have to have previous examples, but as you explore and experiment, you can create your own paradigms as you go.

DANIEL GOLEMAN: Your Holiness, you said one way to do this is by creating a compassionate environment. What might that mean in a medical school? Are there specific attitudes or techniques that would be skillful to introduce to medical students?

COMPASSION AS A NATURAL PART OF LIFE

DALAI LAMA: I believe that human affection is the basis or foundation of human nature. Without that, you can't get satisfaction or happiness as an individual; and without that foundation, the whole human community can't get satisfaction either. In my day-to-day thinking, I always take into account the entire environment, the whole community. Technicians, scientists, doctors, lawyers, politicians, even military personnel and religious people—all these are branches of the human community. So all are basically human beings, and each individual profession is essentially meant for humanity, isn't it? It is supposed to serve humanity, so all these different human activities start with that motivation to do something for our own community. At the very least, one aims to benefit one's own family. Even this very limited community has altruism at its root. All these different human activities start from that motivation, and these activities are meant for humanity. Therefore the basic human condition, or human quality, is human affection. That's the key thing, right?

It is possible to develop, or promote, that human quality, because human nature, I believe, is basically compassionate. Of course, as I mentioned earlier, anger, hatred, and all these negative emotions are also part of the human mind. However, the dominant force of the human mind still is compassion.

Conception takes place when a male and female come together, due, I think, to genuine love. That means they respect each other, are concerned with each other, and share a sense of responsibility. It's not like the situation we discussed the other day, in which sexual intercourse takes place because of other things. These other cases are really mad love. There is, I think, mad desire for sexual pleasure, and these negative things develop. But proper human sexuality, according to a kind of natural law, I think includes some sense of responsibility. In that way, human life begins. Then during those few months in the mother's womb, the mother's state of mind has a strong influence on the development of the child. Then especially during the few weeks after birth, according to scientists, the mother's physical touch is a most important factor for the healthy development of the baby.

I always tell people that a mother is a true teacher of compassion and human affection. Therefore, I do not consider compassion as unique to religion. It's basic human nature that we all share. Mother's milk is, I think, a symbol of compassion. Without mother's milk we cannot survive, so our first act as a baby together with our mother is sucking milk from our mother, or from someone who acts as our mother, with a feeling of great closeness. At that time we may not know how to express what love is, what compassion is, but there is a strong feeling of closeness. From the mother's side also, if there is no strong feeling of closeness toward the baby, her milk may not flow readily. So mother's milk is, I think, a symbol of compassion and human affection.

We have already discussed how illness is very much influenced by states of mind and also the patient's relationship with the doctor. In my own experience, when I visit a doctor, the doctor's smile is very meaningful. A doctor may be a very, very good doctor, a real professional, but if the smile is not there, sometimes I feel slightly uncomfortable. [*laughter*] If the doctor has a genuine smile and takes serious concern, then I feel safe and there is a definite benefit. That's human nature, isn't it? Then, on the last day of our life, in reality it doesn't matter whether you have a friend or not. Very soon you will have to depart from your good friends. Nevertheless, if you are accompanied by some trusted person, even at that moment you feel calm and secure.

Therefore, I think human life is very much based on human affection. As I stated at the beginning, my main concern is that we can explain basic human nature without recourse to any religious system. You scientists are giving me more ammunition now! The modern economy's situation, and also the environment and the population—all these things, I think, are very forceful reminders to us that we should be good human beings; we should work together more cooperatively. During the last few days we have talked much about cells. It seems each individual is a cell, isn't it? This planet is like a human body, and in some sense each of us is a minor component. Without coordination, one individual body cannot be sustained, cannot be healthy, cannot survive. Similarly, the planet can be considered as a human body, and each individual human being is like a cell. Sometimes some cells can become very troublesome! But others can help save the body. That is reality, not just a metaphysical issue.

Scientific progress and discoveries are very much dependent on many factors, economic, political, social, and so forth. The positions taken in scientific fields are not adopted independently. I feel that's really the case. When Western experts become genuine specialists, their field of interest becomes too small. If you are fully involved with a limited topic, this can be problematic. And also sometimes this takes on a destructive nature, because you cannot see the relevance or the negative consequences for the larger interest. Think of the neutron bomb, which kills people in the immediate environment, but does not destroy houses and the like. Later, when the war is finished, then other people can settle in those houses. In contrast, with other weapons there is not only the immediate killing of people, but a lot of other destruction as well, so later people have more hard labor. From that viewpoint, the neutron bomb is "better," but it would be even better yet if we produced some weapon that did not kill those innocent soldiers, but went straight to the generals, or the policy-makers! [*laughter*] That would be best, I think. Without any trouble for these innocent people, let the weapon go to the one person who decided on the war.

So you see, if you look from just one angle, these achievements of awful destructive power can be seen as a great achievement; but then because they bring us disaster, more pain and more suffering, we categorize these things as negative. So again, this has very much to do with basic human feeling.

So that is my approach and my conviction. All individuals, whether scientists, religious practitioners, communists, or extreme atheists—it doesn't matter—all are human beings. All are members of this human community. Everyone has the responsibility to be concerned with the entire community. This is not simply a religious principle, it has to do with one's own self-interest. We do it not for God, not for Buddha, not for some other planet, but for our own planet where we live. It is in our own interest. It's very important to have this kind of perspective and understanding. I have no idea how this should be applied to the medical field in particular. Basically that is the system, the whole structure.

Sometimes I tell people the following example: These different fingers with this palm are very useful. Even one finger can work, but without this palm, no matter how powerful each individual finger is in isolation, it cannot function. Whether the medical field, the religious field, or the scientific field—each of these are useless, and even destructive, when they fail to relate to this theme of our basic humanity. So I say these must be connected with our basic human feeling of affection; then all these different human activities become constructive, don't they?

ABOUT THE CONTRIBUTORS

Francisco Varela, Ph. D., is Director of Research at the National Center for Scientific Research (CNRS), Paris. He is the author of many research articles and eleven books, including *Embodied Mind*.

Clifford Saron, Ph. D., is a psychologist at the Albert Einstein Medical School in New York City.

Richard Davidson, Ph. D., is director of the Laboratory for Affective Neuroscience at the University of Wisconsin.

Daniel Brown, Ph. D., is an assistant clinical professor in psychology at Harvard Medical School. The author of eight books, he has researched meditative traditions for twenty-five years.

Lee Yearley, Ph. D., is a professor of religion at Stanford University. He is the author of *Mencius and Aquinas: Theories and Conceptions of Courage*.

Daniel Goleman, Ph. D., is a contributing science writer to the *New York Times*, and author of *Emotional Intelligence*.

Sharon Salzberg is a principal teacher at the Insight Meditation Society in Barre, Massachusetts. She is the author of *Lovingkindness: The Revolutionary Art of Happiness*.

Jon Kabat-Zinn, Ph. D., is director of the Stress Reduction and Relaxation Program at the University of Massachusetts Medical Center. He is author of *Wherever You Go, There You Are*.

Appendix: About the Mind and Life Institute

R. ADAM ENGLE AND
FRANCISCO J. VARELA

THE MIND AND LIFE dialogues between His Holiness the Dalai Lama and Western scientists were brought to life through a collaboration between R. Adam Engle, a North-American businessman, and Dr. Francisco J. Varela, a Chilean-born neuroscientist living and working in Paris. In 1984 Engle and Varela, who did not know one another at the time, each independently had the initiative to create a series of cross-cultural meetings where His Holiness and scientists from the West would engage in extended discussions over a period of several days.

Engle, a Buddhist practitioner since 1974, had become aware of His Holiness' long-standing, keen interest in science and of his desire to both deepen his understanding of Western science and to share his own understanding of Eastern contemplative science with Westerners. Varela, also a Buddhist practitioner since 1974, had met His Holiness at an international meeting in 1983, as a speaker at the Alpbach Symposia on Consciousness. Their communication was immediate. Their encounter led to a series of informal discussions over the next few years.

In the Autumn of 1984, Engle, with Michael Sautman, met

with His Holiness' youngest brother, Tendzen Choegyal (Ngari Rinpoche), in Los Angeles and presented a plan to create a week-long cross-cultural scientific meeting, provided His Holiness agreed to participate. Rinpoche graciously offered to take the matter up with His Holiness, and within days reported that His Holiness would very much like to engage in discussions with scientists authorizing Engle and Sautman to organize a meeting.

Meanwhile, Dr. Varela was moving forward with his ideas for a meeting, and in the Spring of 1985 a common friend, Dr. Joan Halifax, then director at the Ojai Foundation, suggested that perhaps Engle, Sautman, and Varela could pool their complementary skills and work together to organize an event. The four got together at the Ojai Foundation in October 1985 and agreed to go forward jointly. It was decided to focus on the scientific disciplines dealing with mind and life as the most fruitful of the possible interfaces between science and the Buddhist tradition. "Mind and Life" became the name of the first meeting and, eventually of the Institute itself.

It took two more years of work among Engle, Varela, and the private office of His Holiness before the first meeting was held October, 1987, in Dharamsala, India. During this time, we collaborated closely to find a useful structure for the meeting. Engle took on the job of general coordinator with primary responsibility for fund raising, relations with His Holiness and his office, and all other general aspects of the project, while Francisco, acting as scientific coordinator, took on primary responsibility for the scientific content, invitations to scientists, and editing of meeting transcripts.

This division of responsibility between general and scientific coordinators worked so well that it has been continued throughout all subsequent meetings. To date, Engle has been the general coordinator of all five Mind and Life conferences, and, while Varela has not been the scientific coordinator of all of them, he has always remained a guiding force and Engle's closest partner in the project.

A word is in order here concerning the uniqueness of this series of conferences. The bridges that can be built between

Buddhism and modern life science, in particularly the neuro-sciences, are notoriously difficult to engineer. Varela had a first taste of this when helping to establish a science program at the Naropa Institute, a liberal arts institution created by Tibetan meditation master Chögyam Trungpa Rinpoche. In 1979 the program received a grant from the Sloan Foundation to organize what was probably the very first conference of its kind, "Comparative Approaches to Cognition: Western and Buddhist." Some twenty-five academics from prominent American institutions were brought together from various disciplines: mainstream philosophy, cognitive science (neuro-science, experimental psychology, linguistics, artificial intelligence) and, of course, Buddhist studies. The meeting provided a hard lesson on the care and finesse that the organization of a cross-cultural dialogue requires.

Thus in 1987, profiting from the Naropa experience, and wishing to avoid some of the pitfalls encountered in the past, several operating principles were adopted that have worked extremely well in making the Mind and Life series extraordinarily successful. Perhaps the most important was the decision that scientists would not be chosen solely for their reputations but for their competence in their domain, as well as for their open-mindedness. Some familiarity with Buddhism is helpful, but not essential, so long as a healthy respect for Eastern contemplative science is present.

Next, the curriculum was adjusted as further conversations clarified how much of the scientific background would need to be filled in for His Holiness. To ensure that the meetings would be fully participatory, we structured each of them to begin with a presentation by Western scientists in the morning session. In this way, His Holiness could be briefed on the basic ground of a field of knowledge. The morning presentations were based upon a broad, mainstream, nonpartisan, scientific point of view. The afternoon session was devoted solely to the discussion that naturally flowed from the morning presentation. During this discussion session, the morning presenter could state his or her personal preferences and judgments, if they differed from the generally accepted viewpoints.

The issue of translation within meetings posed a significant challenge, as it was literally impossible to find a Tibetan native fluent in both English and science. This challenge was overcome by setting up a team of two wonderful interpreters, one Tibetan and one a Westerner with a scientific background, placing them next to one another during the meeting. This allowed the quick, on-the-spot clarification of terms that was absolutely essential. Thubten Jinpa, a Tibetan Monk then studying for his Geshe degree at Ganden Shartse monastery and now at Cambridge University; and Alan Wallace, a former monk in the Tibetan tradition with a degree in physics from the University of Massachusetts at Amherst and a Ph.D. in religious studies from Stanford University, interpreted at the first conference and have continued to do so for further meetings. During Mind and Life V, when Dr. Wallace was unavailable, the Western interpreter was Dr. José Cabezon.

A final principle that has contributed to the success of the Mind and Life series has been that the meetings have been conducted entirely in private: no press, no television cameras, few invited guests have been allowed to observe. This stands in sharp contrast to meetings in the West where the public stature of the Dalai Lama makes a relaxed, spontaneous discussion virtually impossible. The Mind and Life Institute records the meetings on videotape and audiotape for archival purposes and transcription, but the actual meeting remains protected in order to facilitate exploration.

The curriculum for the first Mind and Life dialogue introduced various broad themes from cognitive science touching on scientific method, neurobiology, cognitive psychology, artificial intelligence, brain development, and evolution. In attendance were Jeremy Hayward, physics and philosophy of science; Robert Livingston, neuroscience and medicine; Eleonor Rosch, cognitive science; Newcomb Greenleaf, computer science; and Francisco Varela, neuroscience and biology.

The event was an enormously gratifying success in that

both His Holiness and the participants felt that there was true meeting of minds with some substantial advances. The Dalai Lama encouraged us to continue with further dialogues on a biannual basis, a request that we were only too happy to honor. Mind and Life I was transcribed, edited, and published as *Gentle Bridges: Conversations with the Dalai Lama on the Sciences of Mind* edited by Jeremy Hayward and Francisco J. Varela (Boston: Shambala Publications, 1992). This book has been translated into French, Spanish, German, Japanese, and Chinese.

Mind and Life II took place in October 1989 in Newport, California, with Robert Livingston as the scientific coordinator and with the emphasis on brain sciences. It was a two-day event, whose focus was more specifically on neuroscience. Invited were Patricia S. Churchland, philosophy of science; J. Allan Hobson, sleep and dreams; Larry Squire, memory; Antonio Damasio, neuroscience; and Lewis Judd, mental health. The event was made especially memorable when His Holiness was awarded the Nobel Peace Prize on the first morning of the meeting.

With Mind and Life III in 1990, the conference returned to Dharamsala. Having organized and attended both the first two conferences, Adam Engle and Tenzin Geyche Tethong agreed that have the meetings in India produced a much better result than holding them in the West did. Daniel Goleman (psychology) served as the scientific coordinator for Mind and Life III, which focused on the theme of the relationship between emotions and health. Participants included Daniel Brown, experimental psychology; Jon Kabat-Zinn, medicine; Clifford Saron, neuroscience; Lee Yearley, philosophy; and Francisco Varela, immunology and neuroscience. The material from Mind and Life III makes up the present volume.

During Mind and Life III, a new arena of exploration emerged that went beyond the format of the conferences, but served as their natural extention: Clifford Saron, Richard Davidson, Francisco Varela, and Gregory Simpson initiated a project to investigate the effects of meditation on long-term meditators. The idea was to profit from the good will and trust that had been built with the Tibetan community in Dharamsala and the willingness of His Holiness for this kind of research. We then decided to create a Mind and Life Network, linking up other scientists interested in research on topics relating Eastern contemplative experience and Western science. With seed money from the Hershey Family Foundation, we formed the nonprofit organization called the Mind and Life Institute, which has chaired by Engle since its inception. The Fetzer Institute funded two years of expenses for the network and for the initial stages of the research project. A progress report was submitted to the Fetzer Foundation in 1994; as work continues in publishing many of the project conclusions, work also continues on various related aspects such as attention and emotional response.

Mind and Life IV took place in October 1992 with Francisco Varela again acting as scientific coordinator. The topic and title for the dialogue was "Sleeping, Dreaming, and Dying." Invited participants were Charles Taylor, philosophy; Jerome Engel, medicine; Joan Halifax, anthropology and death and dying; Jayne Gackenbach, psychology of lucid dreaming; and Joyce McDougal, psychoanalysis. The account of this conference is now available as *Sleeping, Dreaming and Dying: Dialogues with the Dalai Lama,* edited by Francisco Varela (Boston: Wisdom Publications, 1997).

Mind and Life V was held in Dharamsala in October 1994. The topic was "Altruism, Ethics, and Compassion," and the scientific coordinator was Richard Davidson. In addition to Dr. Davidson, participants included Nancy Eisenberg, child development; Robert Frank, altruism in economics; Anne Harrington, history of science; Elliott Sober, philosophy; and Ervin Staub, psychology and group behavior. The volume covering this meeting is in preparation.

Mind and Life VI is planned for October 1997. It will be held in Dharamsala again, and, for the first time the topic will shift from the biological sciences to physics and cosmology. Arthur Zajonc is the scientific coordinator and Adam Engle will once again be the general coordinator.

Over the years, the institute has been supported by the generosity of several individuals and organizations. Barry and Connie Hershey of the Hershey Family Foundation joined our support group in 1990 and have become the Institute's most loyal and steadfast patrons. Their support has not only made the conferences possible, but has also brought the Institute itself to life. Over the years we have also received generous support from the Fetzer Institute, the Nathan Cummings Foundation, Mr. Branco Weiss, Adam Engle, Michael Sautman, Mr. and Mrs. R. Thomas Northcote, Ms. Christine Austin, and Mr. Dennis Perlman. On behalf of His Holiness the Dalai Lama and all the other participants over the years, we humbly thank all of these individuals and organizations. Your generosity has had a profound impact on the lives of many people.

We would also like to thank a number of people for their assistance in making the work of the Institute a success over the years. Many of these people have assisted the work of the Institute since the beginning, and we are very grateful for their participation. We thank and acknowledge His Holiness the Dalai Lama, Tenzin Geyche Tethong and the other wonderful people of the private office of His Holiness, Ngari Rinpoche and Rinchen Khandro together with the staff of the Kashmir cottage, all the scientists, scientific coordinators, and interpreters, Maazda Travel in the United States and Middle Path Travel in India, Pier Luigi Luisi, Elaine Jackson, Clifford Saron, Zara Houshmand, Alan Kelly, Peter Jepson, Pat Aeilo, Thubten Chodron and Laurel Chiten, Shambala Publications, and Wisdom Publications.

The Mind and Life Institute was created in 1990 as a 50Ic3 public charity to support the Mind and Life dialogues and to promote cross-cultural scientific research and understanding. We can be reached at P.O. Box 94, Boulder Creek, CA 95006. Telephone (408) 338-2123; fax: (408) 338-3666; E-mail: aengle@engle.com.

INDEX

Abhidharma system: absence of fear, 172; ignorance, 39; restlessness, 38

action: consequences of, 25; doing and nondoing, 123; equilibrium and, 87; unwholesome, 170-171, 202, 203. *See also* behavior; karma

Ader, Robert, 56

affection (human), 29, 30, 246–247, 250

afflictions. *See* mental afflictions

afterlife, 16, 17

aggression, 191

agitation. *See* stress

altruism, 202, 246–247; in animals, 27, 28; ethics and, 19; in physicians, 245

amygdala, 78–79

anatman, 111, 144n1

anger: afflictive nature of, 30, 34; Buddhist view, 81–82, 88, 171, 173–175; as Christian vice, 167; clinical studies on, 34, 35–37; cultural aspects, 188; headaches and, 152; psychological view, 70, 188; self-directed, 189, 190, 191, 196; stress reduction and, 135, 137

animals: altruism in, 27, 28; and humans compared, 43, 93, 167, 214–215

antibodies, 51, 52, 53; classical view, 54–55; experiments with, 65

antidotes, 190, 197

anxiety, 128–129; in affluent society,

185; anticipatory, 92; Cognitive Somatic Anxiety questionnaire, 128; stress reduction program and, 135, 137; visual perception and, 221. *See also* stress

apathy, 167–168, 201

approach behavior, 69–71; brain and, 75–76; emotions as, 82, 85

Aquinas, Thomas, 25, 165, 168–170

Aristotle, 25

arthritis, 196

Aryadeva, 175

asthma, 90, 94, 160–161

asymmetry (brain), 75–76

attachment: anger incited by, 174; compassion and, 22, 88; as mental affliction, 81, 82, 171, 172; nonattachment, 122, 123

autoimmune disease: behavioral medicine and, 91; as body's delusion, 66–67; deadly nature of, 64–65, 181; experiments with, 56–57; lupus, 65, 131

autonomic nervous system: amygdala and, 79; body sensation and, 69; dysregulation of, 95, 150; innervation of bone marrow, 57–58; stress and, 90, 92–94, 101

aversion, 69, 186, 238. *See also* withdrawal behavior

awareness: body awareness, 62, 66, 125–126; of breathing, 125, 141; choiceless awareness, 127; of eating, 129; emergence of, 214; emotions and, 216, 238; of former lives, 228, 229; heightened, 232, 233, 234; meaning of, 131, 215, 228; measurement of, 230; in mindfulness meditation, 108, 109, 111, 122, 123; vacillating nature of, 217; in *vipassana* meditation, 112, 238–239. *See also* cognition

balance: in Buddhist ethics, 176; medicine and, 143; self-regulation, 146
Barefoot, John, 35
B-cells, 50, 51–52, 55; experimentation using, 65; immune system and, 53, 54; stress and, 38, 40; vaccines and, 67n1
beginner's mind, 120–123
behavior: approach behavior, 69–71, 75–76, 82, 85; self-regulation, 146; unwholesome, 170–171, 172, 202, 203; wholesome, 172; withdrawal behavior, 68, 69–70, 75, 82, 85
behavioral medicine, 89, 90–91; asthma and, 160–161; headaches and, 149–153; heart disease and, 126–127; hypertension and, 158–160; and technological medicine, 118; treatments, 145–146
Benson, Herbert, 40
bindhu, 231, 232
biofeedback: achieving calm, 40; behavioral medicine and, 89; in specific therapies, 148, 153, 161
biology: basis for ethical system, 67; causes of illness, 91; no perfect state in, 79, 88. *See also* immune system
bliss consciousness, 87
blood flow: control over, 154–155; headaches and, 149, 150; hypertension and, 158; stress and, 94
Bodhisattva: ethics of, 176, 179; and self, 195, 201, 202
body: anxiety in, 128; consciousness and, 212, 228; death process and, 61, 236; and emotion, 69, 84; ethical system of, 34; habits, 146, 160; identity of, 60, 64; and mind, rela-

tionship of, 89, 110, 118, 235; planet analogous to, 248; stress-response cycle, 150; unhealthy attitude towards, 114, 199; visceral learning, 155–158
body awareness, 62, 66, 125–126
body scan, 124–125, 128
Bohm, David, 143
brain: anatomy of, 68, 69, 78–79; awareness, 232; consciousness, 211–213; in death process, 236; emotions and, 68–71; evolution of, 187; immune system and, 56–58; reflexes and, 225; "second brain," 49, 50–52, 65; sensory perception and, 221, 223, 224; stress responses, 57, 93. *See also* brain activity; left brain; right brain
brain activity: consciousness and, 79, 212, 213; emotions and, 71, 213; immune system and, 88; measurement of, 72–73, 219, 239; meditative states and, 238–239; temperament and, 76–78. *See also* left brain; right brain
breathing: awareness of, 124, 125, 129; exercises, 156, 158, 161; in dying process, 236; meditation and, 109, 110, 139, 141, 238; relaxation therapy and, 148; *samatha* and, 112
Buddha: emotions in, 81; killing of Devadatta, 175; teachings of, 116, 175, 227. *See also* buddhas
Buddhadharma, 34, 112
Buddhahood, 20
Buddha nature, 200, 212
buddhas: emotions in, 216; *pratyeka-buddhas*, 202, 207n2
Buddhism: Abhidharma system, 38, 39, 172; afflictive states of mind, 81, 88; availability to non-Buddhists, 113, 127, 204; body awareness, 62, 65; compassion for ignorance, 102–103; concept of self, 60, 193, 194–195, 203; consciousness, 212, 231–232, 236; emotional poles, 69, 85; equanimity, 87–88; karma, 19, 103, 170–

171, 178; lifestyle, 120; Mahayana, 227; Prasangika system, 88, 171, 223; preservation of, 3, 112–113; science and, 6, 227–228, 231–232, 234; three marks of existence, 144n2; in Tibet, 4, 23, 100; virtues and vices in, 170–172. *See also* Theravadin tradition

calm: beneficial emotional state, 34, 40; effect of *vipassana*, 238; in hypertension therapy, 158; mindfulness and, 123, 130; relaxation therapy, 40, 146, 148, 161. *See also* equanimity

cancer, 66, 91

catecholamines, 150, 156

cells: autoimmune disease and, 66–67; individuals analogous to, 248; nerve, 73; receptors, 50–51. *See also* B-cells; T-cells

change: adaptation to, 117, 136; observation of, 109–110

channels *(tsa)*, 231, 232, 233

charity, 170

children: emotions in, 73–75, 187–188; raising, 204–205

choiceless awareness, 127

Christianity: American, 193–194; human nature in, 30; injustice and, 16; Orthodox, 207; virtues and vices in, 166–170

Churchill, Winston, 180

clairvoyance, 228

clear seeing, 114, 123

cognition: and emotion, 69, 83–84, 217, 219; without emotions, 85; of immune system, 54–55; *sems*, 212

cognitive therapy, 197–198; in behavioral medicine, 146, 148–149; low self-esteem and, 204

coherence, 135–156

communication: among cells, 55, 56; between doctor and patient, 142

community: human, 246–247, 249–250; reconnection to, 97–98

compassion: anger and, 173, 174–175; in animals, 28–29, 214; Buddhadharmahood, 112; in Buddhist ethics, 18–20, 22–23, 24, 26; cultivation of, 245–246; in doctors, 142, 245; human nature and, 19, 29, 247; and inequality, 22, 23; mental afflictions and, 88, 171–172; in mindfulness training, 122; stress and, 135; in trauma victims, 102–103; in Western ethics, 11, 15–17, 22. *See also* altruism

confidence: as Christian virtue, 169; lack of, 195; as positive emotion, 34, 41, 83

conscience, 203

consciousness: Buddhist and Western views compared, 211; energies and, 232, 234; preconscious brain activity, 79, 85

sensory perception and, 222–225; subtle degrees of, 6, 212–213, 216, 228, 234; in Tibetan Buddhism, 231–232, 236

contempt: cultural expressions of, 188; self-directed, 196

control (sense of), 41–42, 192

coronary disease, 130

cortex of brain, 68, 69, 78–79, 187

courage, 166, 169

culture: capitalist vs. socialist, 206–207; emotions and, 80–86, 186–187, 188; Eastern European, 207; ethics and, 23–27, 29; facial expressions and, 70–71; low self-esteem and, 189; reconstruction of, 97–98; Tibetan, 184, 205

cynicism, 36

Dalai Lama, 1–2, 100

Darwin, Charles, 70

Davidson, Richard, 69, 219

death: death rates, 42, 43, 45–46; of family member, 117; fear of, 168; process of, 61, 230, 235–236; in scientific studies, 36, 37, 44

delusion, 66–67. *See also* ignorance

depression: clinical studies on, 37–38; and emotions, 34, 75–76; mindfulness meditation and, 135, 139; self-esteem and, 190, 206

despair, 200, 203

destruction: autoimmune disease and,

66–67; human nature and, 30; weapons of, 180–182, 249

de Tocqueville, Alexis, 192

diary, 146, 151, 158

diet, 126

dimensional model of emotions, 71

discrete emotions, 70–71

disease: autoimmune, 56–57, 64–65, 67–68, 91, 181; emotions and, 34; lack of inner balance, 133; scientific studies and, 44. *See also* illness

doctors: compassion in, 142, 245; stress in, 142, 143

doubt, 81, 82

dreams: nightmares of torture victims, 100, 101; subtle consciousness and, 230; of trauma victims, 99

drops *(bindhu)*, 231, 232

Duchenne of Bologne, 74

dyslexia, 57–58

eating meditation, 129

education. *See* learning

EEG, 44, 45, 72, 76, 78

effectors, 53

ego: *anatman,* 111, 144n1; egotism and emotions, 216; negative and positive, 201

Ehrlich, Paul, 55

Ekman, Paul, 70, 72, 84, 188

electroencephalograph (EEG), 44, 45, 72, 76, 78

electromyograph, 153

embarrassment, 188

emotions: body parts and, 124–125; Buddhist terms for, 81, 86; components of, 84; definition of, 69, 85–86; stored emotional pain, 126; unwholesome, 77–78, 85, 88; wholesome, 40–44, 77–78, 85, 88

empathy, 142

emptiness: Buddhist concept, 88, 110, 112, 171; and Western notions compared, 200–201

energy *(lung* or *prana),* 231; in dying process, 235–237; heightened awareness and, 233, 234

Engle, Adam, 2

enlightenment, 22

environment: compassionate, 246; as factor for health, 34, 147, 218; stress and, 95

envy, 167

equanimity: in doctors, 142; health benefits of, 40; lacking in Western systems, 85, 184; as nature of mind, 87; wrathful deities and, 174

equilibrium: disturbance of, 87; emotions and, 80; meaning of, 88; mental afflictions and, 171

ergot, 153

escape reflexes, 52–53

ethics: biology as basis for, 67; Buddhist, 24, 26, 176–177; compassion and, 18–24; culture and, 23–27; nonreligious basis for, 17–18, 21, 28, 44, 244; universal basis for, 28–31, 249–250; virtue and, 11; weapons of destruction, 180–183; Western, 12, 21, 24–25, 26

evil, 30–31, 172

evolution: awareness and, 214; of brain, 187

exercise, 95, 126

existence: cycle of, 103; three marks of, 111, 112, 144n2

eye, 223. *See also* visual perception

facial expression: culture and, 188; emotions and, 69; in newborn babies, 74; studies on, 70–71, 72, 84

faith, 169–170

family, 29, 246

fantasizing: stress and, 96; visceral learning and, 157

fear: amygdala and, 79; in Buddhist tradition, 172–173; of death, 168; as discrete emotion, 70; early childhood emotion, 188; nuclear weapons and, 180; overcoming, 169; right brain and, 68, 69

feelings: being cut off from, 114; difficulty in measuring, 86; and "emotions," 81, 86; in paralyzed people, 84–85. *See also* emotions

fight-or-flight reaction, 89, 93, 130

Fox, Nathan, 74
freedom: and compassion, 16, 88; in ethics, 17–18
Friedman, Howard, 39
friendliness, 42–43

gender: chronic pain and, 137–138; in literature, 186; risk of heart attacks, 37
Gentle Bridges (ed. Varela and Hayward), 3, 7n1
gloom, 218
gluttony, 166–167
God: Christian view, 168, 169, 170; ethics without, 17, 249; as judge, 193; and religion, 29–30
Goleman, Daniel, 128
greed, 168
Guhyasamaja-tantra, 125
guilt, 188, 189, 207

habits learning of, 146–147, 160; unhealthy, 34, 90; visceral learning and, 155, 158
happiness: and brain activity, 68, 75, 77–78; desire for, 170, 194–195; as emotion, 69, 70, 188; human nature and, 246; positive effect of, 34, 43–44; self-contempt and, 189
harmony of body, 88, 127, 133
hatha yoga, 127
hatred. *See* anger
headaches: behavioral medicine and, 90, 149–153; migraine, 150; stress and, 94; visceral learning and, 155–158
health: brain activity and, 80; emotions and, 33, 40–44; limitation of Western view, 237; meaning of, 4, 115, 126. *See also* illness
heart disease: anger and, 35–37; behavioral medicine and, 126–127; depression and, 38; recovery from, 196; reduction in, 138
heart rate, 93, 94, 238
heightened awareness, 232, 233, 234
hemisphere. *See* left brain; right brain
heredity, 34

high blood pressure, 90, 138, 158–160
hope, 169–170
hormones: beta-endorphins, 58; body's wisdom and, 64; emotions and, 69; glucocorticoids, 57; right brain and, 80, 88; testosterone, 37
hostility. *See* anger
human beings: and animals compared, 28, 43, 93, 167, 214–215; human community, 246, 249–250; ideal, 13. *See also* ethics
human nature, 29–30, 189, 246
human rights: culture and, 23; ethical systems and, 16, 20; Western rationalism and, 14, 32n3
hypertension, 90, 138, 158–160
hypnosis, 89, 148

identity: *anatman,* 111, 141n1; body's, 52–53, 59, 64; designated self, 60, 193. *See also* self-esteem
ignorance: evil as, 30–31, 102–103; as mental affliction, 81, 88; and repression, 39; sensory perception and, 223
illness: behavioral medicine and, 90–92; gender and, 37, 137; meaning of, 4, 126; measurement of, 45–46; stress leading to, 89, 95. *See also* disease; health
immune system: basis for ethical system, 33–34; bodily sensation and, 62; brain activity and, 78, 80, 88; communication within, 54; death and, 235; effect of mental states, 34–35, 38–39; measurement of, 45; and nervous system compared, 51–53, 55–56; peripheral and central, 55–56; as "second brain," 49, 50–52, 65
immunology, 53, 55, 65
immunotransmitters, 57
imprisonment, 96, 99–104
individualism, 11, 12–13, 15, 24, 176
information processing, 219–222
inner life: of immune system, 53, 55; trust in, 121
insomnia, 146–147

interdependence: Buddhist notion, 24, 110, 171; of reflexes, 224–225
"intrinsic awareness' (*Rigpa*), 212
irritable bowel syndrome, 94

Jackson, John Hughlings, 70
James, William, 112, 233
joy. *See* happiness
justice, 168–169

Kalachakra-tantra, 233
Kant, Immanuel, 14, 25, 32n3
karma, 32n2; killing and, 178; mental afflictions and, 170–171; and motivation, 19; suffering and, 103
Keller, Helen, 194
killing: justification for, 175–176, 178–179; suicide, 143, 177
kleshas. See mental afflictions
knowledge: awareness and, 232; immune system and, 50; lack of, 16, 18
Kuhn, Thomas, 226

Lama Vairochana, 4
language: of cells, 59; and emotions, 184, 186, 193; of universal truths, 27
learning: at cellular level, 52, 55; habits, 146–147, 160; medical training, 142–143, 245; visceral, 155–158
LeDoux, Joseph, 77
left brain: amygdala and, 79; in children, 73–75; 77; information processing, 219; positive feelings and, 68, 70; temperament and, 77–78
lifestyle: illness related to, 126–127; life-change stress, 94–95
limbic system, 57, 68
listening skills, 142
Locke, John, 32n3
lotus posture, 124
love: discovery of, 199–200; praise and, 204; self-love, 198
loving-kindness (*metta*): as beneficial emotional state, 34, 44; and Christian charity compared, 170; therapy for self-esteem, 189, 191

lupus, 65, 131
lymphocytes, 50; activated and resting, 56, 57; death process and, 61; hormones produced by, 57, 58

Madhyamika Prasangika system, 88, 171, 223
Mahayana Buddhism, 227
mantra: in psychotherapy, 197–198; in *samatha*, 112
Marxism, 21
McClelland, David, 137
measurement: of anxiety, 128; of connectedness, 136–137; of emotions, 71, 85–86; of personality factors, 135–136, 138; problematics in, 45–46, 62; self-monitoring, 151; sense-of-coherence scale, 136
medicine: Buddhist, 234, 245; defense immunology and, 65; and "meditation," 143; psychosomatic, 91. *See also* behavioral medicine
meditation: awareness and, 217; brain activity during, 238–239; in Buddhist tradition, 4, 212, 231; health benefits of, 40, 89; incomplete view of, 113, 123; in relaxation therapy, 148. *See also* mindfulness meditation
memory: of body, 52; cells and, 55; of trauma victims, 99, 101
mental afflictions (*kleshas*), 81, 88; cognition and, 86; equilibrium and, 87; karma and, 170–171; object of anger, 175
mind: afflictions (*kleshas*), 81; anxiety in, 128; discovery of life of, 125; health and, 34, 35, 118; immune system as, 33–34; improvement of, 136; interdependence and, 110; nature of, 87; positive states of, 40–44
Mind and Life Conferences, 1, 2–4, 227
mindfulness meditation: clinical uses, 113–117, 138–140; described, 108–109, 111, 124–131; low self-esteem and, 191, 196; medical effects of, 134–137; principles taught

in, 120–123; in West, 107. *See also* stress reduction and relaxation program

mindfulness training, 116, 117–120, 157; awareness and, 217; and medical training, 142–143. *See also* mindfulness meditation

moderation, 169

mood shifts, 218

mortality. *See* death rates motion: mindfulness of, 127; mobility, 215

motivation: in Buddhist ethics, 19, 26; oneness motive, 136–137; for violence, 177, 180

murder. *See* killing

muscles: and autonomic nervous system, 93, 94; facial, 74; headaches and, 153; relaxation techniques, 148, 149, 150

mutes, 194

myasthenia gravis, 46, 65, 67n2

neocortex, 78–79

nervous system: awareness and, 214; death and, 235; and immune system compared, 51–53, 55–56; mobility and, 215. *See also* autonomic nervous system

network immunology, 55

neurons, 51, 57, 61

neuroscience, 59, 85, 214

nonattachment, 122, 123

nondoing, 115, 120, 123

nonjudgment, 120–121, 122

numbing, 96, 101

oneness motive, 136–137

optimism, 34, 40–41

original sin, 30–31, 167, 193

pain: behavioral medicine and, 90, 146, 157; gender and, 137–138; stress-response cycle and, 150

panic disorders, 138–139

paralysis, 84–85

patience, 120–121

perception: sensory, 216, 222–225; skillful internal, 148; visual, 216,

223, 232, 235; yogic, 231, 232, 234, 237

perfection: Buddhist model, 18; no perfect biological state, 79, 88

perfectionism, 13; Buddhism and, 24, 176; religious belief and, 20; universal, 10, 26, 31; Western ethics and, 11, 12, 15, 24

personality factors, 135–136, 138

plants, 60, 62–63, 214

pleasantness: in dimensional model of emotions, 71; mindfulness of, 129–130. *See also* unpleasantness

positive emotions, 77–78

posttraumatic stress disorder (PTSD), 90, 100, 103–104

praise, 197, 198, 199

Prasangika system: mental afflictions, 88, 171; visual perception, 223

pratyekabuddhas, 202, 207n2

pride, 81, 83, 168

problem solving, 131

psoriasis, 140–141

psychology: child development, 187–188; doubt, 82–83; emotions, 69, 70, 85; social connection, 42. *See also* behavior

psychoneuroimmunology, 49–50, 58; body's identity, 60; first experiments in, 56

psychotherapy: and self-esteem, 195, 197–198, 201–202; trauma victims and, 98

PTSD, 90, 100, 103–104

pulmonary disease, 139–140

rationalism, 13–14; Buddhism and, 24, 176; Western ethics and, 11, 12, 17, 25, 31

reason, 13, 14

receptors (cells), 50, 56, 57

recovery: belief and, 196; depression and, 37

reflexes, 52–52, 224–225

relativity (ethics), 25

relaxation therapy, 40, 146, 148, 161; relaxation program, 115, 116, 117–120, 130

religion: basis for, 29–30; ethics and,

11, 13, 17–18, 27, 244; trauma victims and, 101–102. *See also* Buddhism; Christianity

repression: of anger, 152; of emotional pain, 126; illness and, 39; stress and, 96

responsibility: of all human beings, 249; of scientists, 182–183; sexuality and, 247

rest: equanimity and, 87; stress and, 94

restlessness: *See* stress

retina, 222, 224

right brain: in children, 73–75, 77; depression and, 75–76; emotions and, 68, 73, 80, 88; information processing, 219–220; temperament and, 77–78; withdrawal behavior and, 70

rights. *See* human rights

routines, 95

saccharides, 149

sadness, 37, 70, 188

samadhi, 231, 232, 233

samatha, 111–112, 144n3, 238

samsara, 103

schizophrenics, 229

Schwartz, Gary, 39

science: Buddhism and, 3–4, 6; ethics and, 181–182; limitations of, 229–230; neuroscience, 59, 214; progress in, 248–249

"second brain," 49, 50–52, 65

self: constitution of, 54; identity of, 52, 202; immune system and, 60. *See also* ego

self-centeredness, 194–195

self-confidence, 200, 201, 203

self-esteem: depression and, 206; increase in, 197; therapies for, 191–196, 204; in Tibetan culture, 184–185; in West, 190–192, 201–202, 205–207

self-interest, 195, 249

self-love, 198

self-monitoring: in asthma therapy, 160; in behavioral medicine, 146; of headaches, 151

sensation: emotion and, 69; and immune system, 63; mindfulness training and, 108, 124, 126, 127

sense-of-coherence scale, 136

senses, 212, 233

sensory perception: Buddhist view, 216; and consciousness, 222–225

sexual abuse, 96

sexuality, 166, 247

shame, 188

Shantideva, 172

shravaka, 202, 207n1

silence, 120

simplicity, 116

sins, 166–168, 179

sitting meditation, 125, 128

skepticism, 81

smoking, 147

society: inequality in, 21; lack of connectedness, 192; science and, 181–182; social contact, 42–43; in Western ethics, 13, 17

somatization, 135, 137

speech: information processing, 219; tantric realization and, 233

Spiegel, David, 42

standing meditation, 129, 140

stillness, 113–114

stress, 89, 116–117; as afflictive state, 34; and autonomic nervous system, 92–94; brain's response, 57; change and, 117, 136; clinical studies on, 38–39; coping with, 90, 96; in hospital personnel, 116, 142, 143; illness linked to, 140, 149, 150, 161; mindfulness training for, 130; personality factors and, 135–136, 138; posttraumatic stress disorder, 90, 100, 103–104; social, 95; types of, 94–95

stress reduction and relaxation program: described, 115, 116, 117–120, 130; for medical students, 143; results of, 134–137, 141

stress-response cycle, 150, 156

suffering: compassion and, 18, 23, 171; freedom from, 170; karma and, 103; in mindfulness training, 113, 142; as spiritual opportunity, 100; Western view of, 17

suicide, 143, 177
Sutras: heightened awareness in, 233; *Satipatthana-sutra*, 112, 116

Tantras, 4; *Guhyasamaja-tantra*, 125; *Kalachakra-tantra*, 233; violence in, 173–175
tantric realization, 232
T-cells (Thymal cells), 50; autonomous nervous system and, 58; decrease in, 38; immune system and, 51, 54; increase in, 40, 44; as measurement, 45
temperament, 76–78
therapy. *See* cognitive therapy; relaxation therapy
Theravadin tradition, 144n3; ethics and, 18; loving kindness (*metta*), 189; meditation, 107, 113–117, 129
thought: low self-esteem and, 196–197; meditation and, 109, 110–111, 127, 141; preceding headaches, 156–157; rationalism and, 26; rest and, 87. *See also* cognition
torture, 99–104
tranquility, 87, 172. *See also* equanimity
trauma: posttraumatic stress disorder, 90, 100, 103–104; reactions to, 99–104; treatment of, 96–99
treatment. *See* recovery; therapy
trust: affiliative, 137; mindfulness and, 120, 121
truth: language for, 27; science and, 229

"universal ground" (*Kun shi*), 212
unpleasantness: brain as censor, 219–221; emotions as, 71; mindfulness and, 130–131. *See also* pleasantness
unwholesome behavior: karma and, 170–171; mental afflictions and, 172; refrain from, 202, 203
unwholesome emotions, 85, 88–89

vaccines, 53, 66n1
Vajra recitation, 125

Vajrayana, 233
vanity, 167
Varela, Francisco, 2–3
violence: avoidance of, 177; low self-esteem and, 191; in *Vinaya*, 176–177; in wrathful deities, 173–175
vipassana: brain activity during, 238; practice of, 111–112, 129, 144n4
virtue: Aquinas's list, 168–170; Buddhist view, 4, 170; characteristics of, 165–166; dying process and, 237; and ethics, 11; fear of evil as, 171
visceral learning, 155–158
visualization: in behavioral medicine, 155, 157, 161; Buddhist and non-Buddhist practices compared, 125; of negative emotion, 174; in psoriasis therapy, 140; trauma victims and, 99; and Western ethics, 21
visual perception: in Buddhist psychology, 216, 223; in dying process, 235; information processing, 219, 221–222; low-level vision, 222–223; tantric realization and, 232
vulnerability, 168

warming exercises, 158
weapons of destruction, 180–182
wellness enhancement, 91
wholeness: and health, 115, 143; limits of Western view, 237; negative thoughts and, 199–200
wholesome emotions, 40–44, 85, 88, 172
Williams, Redford, 36
wisdom: of body and mind, 64, 115; Buddhist view, 19–20, 112; as Christian virtue, 168; mindfulness training and, 118, 122
withdrawal behavior: brain and, 68, 75; emotions as, 69–70, 82, 85. *See also* approach behavior

yoga, 126, 127, 128
yogic perception: clear-light state and, 237; of energies, 231, 234; limitations of, 232, 234